Table of Contents

HEALING
WAYS

An Integrative Health Sourcebook

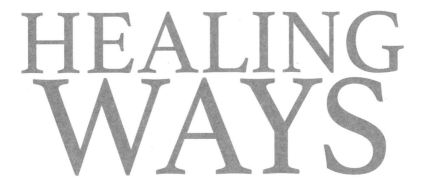

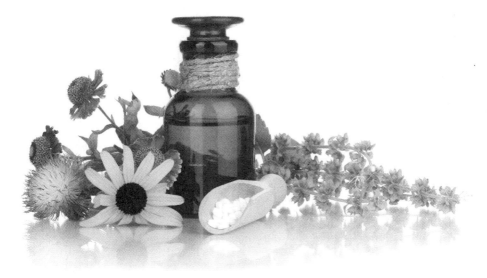

MATILDE PARENTE, M.D., F.C.A.P.

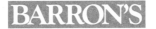

BARRON'S

COVER CREDITS
Fotolia: Monet: front cover (top left); pat_hastings: front cover (top right); Gelpi: front cover (middle).
Shutterstock: Tyler Olsen: front cover (top center); Freya-photographer: front cover (bottom); Africa Studio: back cover and title page.

PHOTO/ILLUSTRATION CREDITS
Gabriella Ritts: 85 (top, bottom)
Shutterstock: Tom Wang: 80; Doglikehorse: 83; Luna Vandoome: 104; Valua Vitaly: 120; lightwavemedia: 128; Sofiaworld: 171; Jezper: 186.

All inquiries should be addressed to:
Barron's Educational Series, Inc.
250 Wireless Boulevard
Hauppauge, New York 11788
www.barronseduc.com

Library of Congress Catalog Card No. 2015004196

ISBN: 978-1-4380-0637-6

Library of Congress Cataloging-in-Publication Data
Parente, M. (Matilde)
Healing ways : an integrative health sourcebook / Matilde Parente, MD, FCAP.
pages cm
Includes index.
ISBN 978-1-4380-0637-6 (paperback)
1. Alternative medicine—Popular works. 2. Self-care, Health. I. Title.
R733.P34   2016
613—dc23   2015004196

Printed in Canada
9 8 7 6 5 4 3 2 1

1

Introduction

IN 1993, A STUDY APPEARED IN THE *NEW ENGLAND JOURNAL OF MEDICINE* THAT jolted mainstream American medicine, rocking prestigious medical centers and small-town country doctors alike. In that special article titled "Unconventional Medicine in the United States," David M. Eisenberg, M.D., and colleagues reported that in the past year, one in three people in their telephone interview study had used at least one unconventional therapy—defined in their study as methods or interventions that were not generally taught at U.S. medical schools at the time or that were not typically available at most U.S. hospitals.

Although methods such as chiropractic, Chinese medicine, massage, and other therapies had long been used across the country, the report shed light on the huge yet underappreciated impact of unconventional care on the American health-care system, which surprised the conventional medical community. By putting numbers on the rate, costs, and use of such care, the study's importance was not lost on academic leaders, the government, health organizations, and the business community.

Just more than two decades later, complementary and alternative medicine practices have assumed an important role in American health care, where they are now increasingly known as **integrative health** or integrative care. The changes have been so swift that in December 2014, the National Center for Complementary and Alternative Medicine (NCCAM), established by Congress in 1998, changed its name to the National Center for Complementary and Integrative Health (NCCIH).

Prompting the name change was the finding that complementary and alternative practices had become such an integral and common aspect of contemporary health care that they were no longer being perceived as "alternative." This new viewpoint is not only shared by the millions of Americans who use such care but is also increasingly held by medical providers of many stripes, including a growing number of medical doctors (M.D.s).

Alternative Medicine: Truly Alternative or "Hidden Mainstream"?

Five years after the 1993 study, Eisenberg and another group of colleagues reported on trends involving the use of certain alternative medicine practices from 1990–97 in a 1998 article published in the *Journal of the American Medical Association*. They reported that the use of the 16 therapies originally studied had jumped from about 33% of the people surveyed to 42% over those seven years. By extending their survey data to the overall U.S. population, the authors offered the then-shocking conclusion that the nearly 50% increase in visits to alternative practitioners was, in total, actually greater than the total number of visits paid to *all* primary care physicians in the country. Moreover, the total out-of-pocket spending on alternative therapies in 1997 was estimated to be about the same as the forecasted out-of-pocket payments made for services by *all* U.S. primary care physicians in that year.

Today, in an unprecedented turnaround, the Consortium of Academic Health Centers for Integrative Medicine lists 63 integrative medicine programs that are affiliated with U.S. medical schools in 25 states, plus the District of Columbia, with more projected to come online in the coming years.

However, despite their widespread use and growing acceptance, many questions regarding nonmainstream health-care methods remain unresolved or under debate. Finding answers to what does and does not work, and which methods might be best for a given illness or condition, can be challenging. Besides, although many integrative methods have histories that trace back thousands of years, questions still linger about certain aspects of safety, effectiveness, or the usefulness of certain methods in various states of health and disease.

PURPOSE AND GOALS

This book aims to revisit and stimulate this conversation. In these pages are ways to help you navigate among different complementary and alternative methods, many of which form the basis of health care for much of the world. Today, many of these therapies have been or are being brought under the umbrella of integrative health— that is, healing methods that may borrow from different unconventional practices in tandem with the advances and practices derived from mainstream medical care. Integrative care is now commonly encountered at leading academic medical centers, community hospitals, and small-group settings, and increasingly in hospice and military care. In less than a generation, integrative care has made enormous strides, claiming its place at the table in discussions of health and wellness on a national and international level.

Yet, despite the surge in popularity of different treatments and supplements, the level or amount of evidence for these therapies and methods has lagged behind their use. This book will introduce you to some of these findings. Much evidence continues to be built and, like many other knowledge areas about health and disease, is very much a work in progress. Expect more changes, discoveries, exceptions, and turnarounds to come as we dig deeper, look harder, and attempt to refine efforts toward safer, effective, and better-informed healing.

HOW TO BENEFIT FROM THIS BOOK

This book aims to provide you with different ways to learn about or to further explore the therapies that interest you most. Although it is designed to present an orderly view of integrative health from the general to the more specific, readers who are already familiar with many of the methods described may wish to focus first on later chapters about methods that serve their specific interests, returning to earlier chapters at another time. Even after you've finished reading the book, you may find yourself returning to the Method Finder section in Chapter 14 to help you address other health concerns. You may wish to add your own notes as new knowledge comes online or when reevaluating certain methods depending on your health status or the experiences you encounter with integrative methods.

HOW TO NAVIGATE THIS BOOK

Chapters 2 through 5 offer a broad overview of various integrative health methods. They also provide important information regarding safety, evidence, different types of practitioners, and how to be a better health-care consumer, regardless of the types of methods you prefer.

Chapters 6 through 10 describe a variety of methods in greater detail and are grouped into chapters on acupuncture and traditional Chinese medicine (6); mind-body approaches and bioenergetics (7); manual therapies and bodywork (8); herbal products and dietary supplements (9); and whole systems of care, such as Ayurveda and homeopathy (10).

Special topics such as cancer, environmental factors, and genetics, among others, are discussed separately in Chapter 11.

Chapter 12 offers information regarding self-care and prevention that will serve most individuals regardless of their health-care preferences or the methods being considered. This is where you will find information about lifestyle, nutrition, weight control, exercise, and healthy habits that go beyond common sense and fads. Prepare to entertain new ideas about wellness and perhaps to consider partnering with your care team in forging new healing ways toward health.

In Chapter 13 you will find a discussion of many myths and misconceptions on both sides of the health-care divide. Read these pages with an open mind, and be ready to entertain possibilities that you might not have considered previously.

Finally, Chapter 14 offers you an important tool, an integrative Method Finder. Use this chart to look up an illness, condition, or method of interest. For example, migraine headache sufferers could consult the finder to zero in on which methods offer the best evidence to date that may merit discussion with their health-care team.

Consult the Glossary at the end of the book to better understand some of the terms used in this book.

Because health information reflects a process that continuously evolves, shifts, and undergoes adjustments, it's important to take the information presented in Chapter 14, as well as that within the other chapters, as works in progress. Understand that the general conditions or methods that appear in Chapter 14 will require further study with respect to your personal situation, whether from this book, other sources, or your health-care team, or on your own. Just because the evidence for a particular method for heart health appears supportive, for example, doesn't necessarily mean it will certainly or always apply to you or to your condition. Personalize the information in this book by establishing open lines of communication with your health-care team to obtain the best possible integrative care.

Many surveys have shown that despite the growing acceptance of nonstandard healing methods, a large number of people still do not tell their providers about their use of other therapies. Moreover, many people who use unconventional care methods tend to use more than one modality. Often, such methods are not being used in a comprehensive way for maximal benefit and safety.

The information in this book may prompt you to ask questions and to learn more about different methods of healing. It is intended to be shared with a qualified health professional and not to be used as medical advice or in place of the advice and care of your health-care team. Chapter 4 provides specific tips to help you follow through in establishing greater communication with your providers about your health preferences, interests, and concerns.

By bringing an array of healing methods to the table, from the level of personal experience to studies involving thousands of patients, we can all help sharpen, broaden, and deepen our knowledge about achieving the best possible health as we pursue the healing ways that will serve us best.

WHERE TO LEARN MORE

Consortium of Academic Health Centers for Integrative Medicine: *www.imconsortium.org*

World Health Organization: *www.who.int*

National Center for Complementary and Integrative Health: *www.nccih.nih.gov*

European Public Health Alliance: *www.epha.org*

2

Integrative Health: An Overview

EWS ABOUT HEALTH GREETS US DAILY. WAVES OF INFORMATION FLOOD OUR inboxes, grab headlines, and flash across our electronic devices. Also chiming in are government leaders; various health organizations; and an endless stream of experts on radio, television, and social platforms.

Amidst the static and noise are some facts, a few theories, and many myths. Altogether, this hodgepodge of information and misinformation can make it difficult to sort through our health options and to choose what's best for us or for our families. The buffet of choices and conflicting opinions can also hinder our ability to navigate our way through the health-care thicket with confidence and knowledge.

The good news is that Americans today have a greater range of health-care choices and information than ever before. This expanding menu of options brings greater empowerment to health consumers in selecting the types of health care that they prefer to receive, the practitioners to help deliver that care, and the self-care methods they wish to pursue.

Along with these new sets of choices come new responsibilities on both sides of the examination table. This new reality has created a growing demand for more information and transparency about what these health choices mean, who is delivering care, and what health consumers can expect from treatments. Consumers and health organizations also want to know about the safety and effectiveness of the available therapies to help them compare, weigh, and choose the best options.

Conventional Western medicine is attempting to adjust to this new reality of heightened health awareness and shifting preferences among health consumers. In some areas of the country, change has been fairly rapid, whereas in other regions, progress in accommodating new ways of looking at health and disease may be slower, or the choices may be more limited.

Regardless of the region, increasing numbers of Americans are becoming interested in the health options offered by a variety of health practices that are often termed (and sometimes dismissed as) complementary and alternative medicine, abbreviated CAM. The concepts and terms preferred in this book are **integrative medicine** and **integrative health**.

TERMS AND CONCEPTS

Various terms have been used to describe or categorize the types of healing methods that differ from the styles of medicine typically practiced in the United States. Complementary, alternative, integrative, and holistic are a few of the most common terms. Other words you may encounter are natural, native, and traditional, among others.

You may be wondering what these terms mean and whether they are describing the same things with respect to treatments and approaches. If they do not, you may be curious about how they differ and how you can find more information that helps you decide which approach appears best for you.

To begin, it helps to first define the Western-based approach to medicine and healing as practiced by most medical doctors who are M.D.s and doctors of osteopathy (D.O.s) in the United States as **mainstream** or **conventional medicine**.

In contrast, other medical or healing systems or beliefs can be viewed as **alternative medicine**. As its name implies, alternative medicine includes approaches that generally fall outside mainstream beliefs or that are used instead of mainstream practices. An example would be a person who does not want to take prescription drugs for cholesterol control and who chooses to use red yeast rice instead.

From a conventional view, many alternative approaches may not have demonstrated an acceptable level of proof or effectiveness—or safety, in some cases—to warrant their use or acceptance. In fact, the quality of many studies examining the uses and usefulness of alternative methods has been highly variable, with varying degrees of proof of effectiveness. Yet, a similar statement could also apply to many of conventional medicine's therapies.

Despite this knowledge gap, attitudes toward alternative methods have undergone a dramatic shift. Many Americans no longer consider therapies such as acupuncture or the use of herbal products as alternative at all. Increasingly, researchers and conventional medical practitioners are becoming more interested in, more informed about, or more accepting of the alternative therapies their patients are choosing.

Complementary medicine is another commonly used term. It refers to practices that may fall outside the mainstream in approach but that are used alongside conventional therapies. An example would be a cancer patient who uses certain supplements or meditation to help them cope with the effects of their cancer or chemotherapy.

Perhaps because alternative medicine seems to imply an either/or choice while complementary medicine involves add-on care options, the term **integrative medicine** has come into wider use among practitioners, organizations, and health consumers.

Integrative medicine extends the concepts of complementary and alternative medicine. Integrative practices aim to personalize care by bringing together treatments that may borrow from both mainstream and alternative approaches in a way that is informed by science, best practices, and evidence. Best integrative practices aim to achieve the best possible outcome in a personalized way, aligning effectiveness, teamwork, safety, and the preferences of the individual.

Integrative methods also take into account lifestyle factors as important aspects of health and wellness. Often, integrative care may involve changing lifestyle choices toward a more healthful, mind-centering, and sustainable path.

Integrative approaches are less concerned about boundaries between various care models and are more focused on healing that is centered on the whole person. Integrative care is interactive, featuring patients or clients who are actively participating in their health together with a cooperative, communicative team of healing professionals. That team may include many types of expertise and different specialists who share a vision of care that is holistic, effective, and safe.

For example, modern cancer care has changed dramatically from a model that was once largely driven by technology and a paternalistic "doctor knows best" mentality. Progressive cancer care increasingly includes services and treatments that not very long ago would have been considered as alternative or perhaps fringe medicine by many mainstream practitioners. Today, more than half of cancer patients use some type of CAM, from acupuncture to **mind-body** relaxation techniques to herbal products and various supplements. Ideally, as examined in Chapter 4, the use of these other methods occurs with the knowledge and involvement of the patients' health-care team members to maximize benefits and minimize potential problems.

Other Common Terms

Functional medicine is a fairly recent term. Developed as a discipline in the 1990s by a Ph.D., functional medicine encompasses a diverse group of practitioners that includes medical doctors and other health-care practitioners from different disciplines such as nutrition and chiropractic.

Functional medicine approaches attempt to assess the whole person in the context of lifestyle, genes, and the environment along with how all these factors may combine to affect health and well-being. Evaluations by functional medicine practitioners often include an array of tests for different types of suspected overgrowths, deficiencies, and toxins. Such testing is somewhat controversial because some of these findings or test results have not been sufficiently proven to implicate actual disease, to fully explain certain symptoms, or to notably affect health outcomes.

Holistic medicine (also spelled as wholistic) is a term used for an approach to healing and wellness that encompasses the whole person—body, mind, and spirit—including a person's emotional state and feelings. Because holistic care is more of a philosophical or individualized approach to healing than a defined system of care, many practitioners and health consumers may have their own definitions or beliefs about what they consider holistic care.

Advocates of mainstream practices may consider some aspects of holistic care as subjective, unscientific, or even potentially risky—at times with good reason. However, the same could also be said of certain treatments and approaches pursued by conventional practitioners.

Within any system of care, health consumers are best served by care that is delivered competently and compassionately, that is informed by reliable data, and that actually delivers or helps to bring about the desired result with the maximum degree of safety. Cost, value, and fiscal responsibility are other elements that warrant consideration.

Natural medicine is another frequently used term, although it is rarely defined with accuracy or consistency. The term "natural" does not carry an established or regulated definition that allows consumers to know exactly what the person, remedy, or therapy attached to the term "natural" means. While natural medicine may refer to the use of natural methods for health issues, "natural" can and does mean different things to different people.

Examples of natural care might include using honey for a skin scrape or the sap from a freshly sliced aloe vera leaf to cool a sunburn. Others might consider over-the-counter herbal supplements or probiotics as examples of natural healing, even though many of these products have been highly processed or altered in some way and may be of questionable potency, purity, or safety. Chiropractors who mainly use manipulation and manual measures in their practice may also consider these methods as natural healing, as might naturopaths or acupuncturists who use energy-stimulating devices. In some instances, "natural" may merely signify prescription drug–free methods.

A less common term is **native** or **traditional medicine**, which generally refers to healing practices or folk remedies that relate to a particular tradition, often within an indigenous culture. Examples include the native healing practices of Native Americans or those of indigenous tribes and cultures such as the Maori of New Zealand or native Hawaiians.

These native or folk healing traditions mostly have been passed down from one generation to the next by word of mouth and mentoring, rather than codified or organized into writings and books. Native practices abound around the world as they have for millennia, forming the foundation of health care for millions of people worldwide. Indeed, some of these practices have contributed mightily to what we now consider modern, mainstream care.

Nature's Medicine Cabinet

For centuries, native and ethnic people who live around the world's equatorial belt have used various medicinal plants to prevent and treat malaria. In colonial times, Spanish priests witnessed a native healing ritual of the Amazon's Quechua tribe for malarial fevers that used the bark of a shrub that was later found to contain quinine, the chemical basis for the first successful anti-malarial medicine. More recently, the Chinese mined its ancient medicine chest to rediscover sweet wormwood, an herbal remedy that was used for malaria in China as far back as the Jin dynasty. Using modern scientific techniques that allowed the extraction of the chemical artemisinin from the herb, the ancient sweet wormwood native plant unlocked the key to a modern remedy that is now used worldwide to help combat a disease that still claims nearly 700,000 lives worldwide each year.

TRADITION: WHOLE SYSTEMS OF CARE

Another set of traditional healing practices relates to cultural values and spiritual beliefs as well as a way of life, often called **whole systems of care**. Examples include traditional Chinese medicine (TCM); other Asian healing traditions such as Japan's Kampo; and Ayurveda, an ancient set of practices associated with modern-day India.

Unlike other types of native traditions that have been passed down as mostly oral history, whole systems of care or ancient healing practices such as TCM and Ayurveda have deep historical and philosophical roots that have also been based on the written word, allowing these practices to be preserved and to evolve over centuries.

For example, Ayurvedic approaches to ways in which illness may affect the natural balance of the body were memorialized two to four centuries BCE in the *Charaka Samhita*, written in Sanskrit. While having a recorded account does not ensure truth or reliability, practitioners who follow these belief systems tailor their practice methods to techniques, formulations, and traditions that have a certain traceability and that have been modified—and hopefully improved—through trial and error over thousands of years and human experiences.

The unique approaches and philosophies behind healing systems such as TCM and Ayurveda are discussed in later chapters.

Part of what makes these types of healing systems so different from conventional medicine is that TCM and Ayurveda, as two prominent examples, view illness in ways that differ greatly from mainstream medicine. Such traditional healing methods approach the person affected by an illness or condition through examination of the balance and interplay of mind-body-spirit, including perhaps diet and bioenergetics, leading to corresponding treatments.

In addition, the word choices and concepts in whole systems of care can differ dramatically from those used by mainstream practitioners. For example, in evaluating a person experiencing bloating or an upset stomach, the words and concepts attached to the balancing of the Ayurvedic elements of Air, Earth, Fire, Space, and Water can seem confusing or might not make a great deal of sense to a mainstream gastrointestinal doctor who is thinking about stomach acid or reflux mechanisms to explain the findings from a different perspective.

WHO USES INTEGRATIVE MEDICINE OR CAM?

Americans are seeking out different methods of care by the millions, whether in tandem with conventional care or on its own. According to 2012 responses to the National Health Interview Survey of nearly 40,000 households, one in three Americans use complementary health methods. The prior 2007 survey found that the rate of CAM use was even higher among people in their fifties. Other studies have reported rates of CAM use among Americans of up to 80%, with higher rates observed among people with certain conditions, such as headache, cancer, or certain types of pain.

Similar to the 2007 findings, the 2012 survey noted that the most frequent complementary approach chosen was the use of supplements other than vitamins and minerals, used by almost one in five adult survey participants and by one in 20 children aged four to 17. Next common were the use of chiropractic or osteopathic care, yoga, massage, meditation, mind-body techniques, and acupuncture, some of which are shown below.

Type of CAM Used in the Past 12 Months

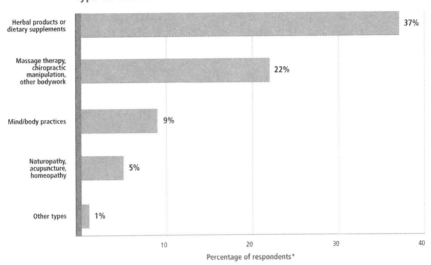

*Base: All respondents (n=1,013). Sampling error: ±3.1 percentage points. Respondents could choose more than one answer.
Source: AARP/NCCAM Survey of U.S. Adults 50+, 2010
Credit: National Center for Complementary and Alternative Medicine, NIH, DHHS

All of this care doesn't come cheaply. Based on figures from the 2007 survey, Americans were spending more than $34 billion yearly on CAM products, services, and visits to various practitioners. While this figure made up less than 2% of all national health-care expenses, it accounted for a whopping 11.2% of all out-of-pocket health-care spending.

Fast forward to 2011, when the U.S. Centers for Disease Control and Prevention (CDC) reported that more than half of all Americans used **dietary supplements**. By 2012, Americans were spending more than $32 billion on dietary supplements alone, nearly eclipsing the total CAM expenditures reported in 2007.

What is driving the increasing use of these integrative therapies? And what does the growth of CAM mean for you, your family, and your community? This book aims to explore many of these questions along with details about the therapies and practitioners themselves.

Can't We All Get Along?

One of the more notable ways in which many integrative practices or alternative medical systems differ from conventional care is in the use of botanical and other natural products. Many mainstream physicians and practitioners are not as likely to prescribe one or many of these products for a variety of reasons, as discussed in detail in Chapters 3 and 9.

Among the most common reasons given by mainstream practitioners for not using botanical or dietary supplements—or for only using a few or only using them in limited ways—is their concern regarding the limited evidence for the effectiveness of many of these products. Another concern regards the safety and reliability of these products. There is also uncertainty regarding the most fitting dose for a given condition or the best available (and affordable) formulation. Many conventional practitioners may be unfamiliar or inexperienced with the use of such products. As one example, a national survey of cancer specialists reported in 2014 that about two-thirds of the oncologists felt unprepared to answer cancer patients' questions about herbs and supplements, with about 60% noting that they hadn't received any training in this field. Recently, however, greater educational opportunities are becoming available to mainstream practitioners regarding the use of supplements and natural products for health.

Why Do People Use CAM?

Health consumers develop their own beliefs or reasons for pursuing self-care or for seeking out an integrative practitioner. Depending on their health status, these reasons might reflect a desire to exercise greater control over their own health, to prevent illness, to boost nutritional or immune status, or to improve overall wellness.

Many people simply prefer a less invasive; less chemical; and more natural, self-healing approach to health that minimizes or avoids prescription drugs. Others may seek treatment for a condition for which conventional care has shortcomings, or for situations in which the available options are unacceptable to the person in need.

All too frequently, CAM is pursued by people who feel that their relationship or communication with their conventional medical provider is lacking in some fundamental or unfixable way.

Some of the reasons for using CAM that were given by people who were age 50 or older, according to a 2010 study, are shown on the next page.

Reasons for CAM Use

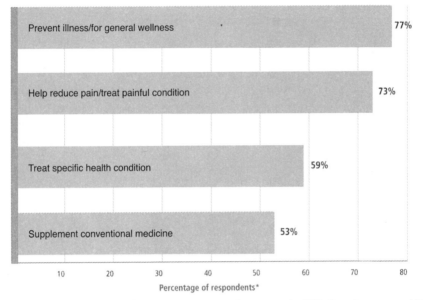

Reason	Percentage
Prevent illness/for general wellness	77%
Help reduce pain/treat painful condition	73%
Treat specific health condition	59%
Supplement conventional medicine	53%

Percentage of respondents*

*Base: Respondents who used CAM in past 12 months or ever (n=539). Sampling error: ±4.2 percentage points. Respondents could choose more than one answer.
Source: AARP/NCCAM Survey of U.S. Adults 50+, 2010.
Credit: National Center for Complementary and Integrative Health, NIH, DHHS.

WHO PRACTICES CAM?

Before examining the varied complementary and alternative approaches, it helps to take a look at who practices CAM and integrative medicine as well as their respective levels of expertise. Do such practitioners receive training that is similar in rigor or scope to that of conventional doctors, and if so, who—if anyone—verifies that training? When training differs from that of mainstream practitioners, how much training is required and in what ways does it differ? Are nonconventional practitioners bound to an oath to practice ethically? Do they maintain their expertise or undergo continuing education, voluntarily or as required? In other words, what kind of doctor is your doctor?

Health-care consumers want and expect answers to these important questions. Consumers, especially those without a background in science or health, deserve to know that the professionals whose care they seek for complex conditions or the practitioners who use advanced testing or equipment in their diagnosis and treatment are adequately trained and qualified to render such care; to interpret complex test results; and to objectively assess the usefulness, safety, and reliability of certain medical devices. Having many degrees and abbreviations appended to a practitioner's name is not enough—consumers also want to know what they mean and what significance they may or may not have to the quality of their care.

Consider your choice of practitioner carefully and wisely—and remain open to reconsidering your choice along your healing path. Keep an open mind about seeking out another opinion from a reliable practitioner who ideally lacks financial conflicts and narrow or rigid viewpoints and, most importantly, has your best interests in mind.

Conventional Medical Doctors

The two main types of mainstream medical doctors you are likely to encounter in the U.S. are M.D.s (doctors of medicine) and D.O.s, (doctors of osteopathy). M.D.s outnumber D.O.s in the U.S. by a ratio of nearly ten to one. Another group of mainstream doctors you may interact with are pharmacists. They are the hidden jewels of conventional care who know a great deal about all types of medicines—both pharmaceutical and, increasingly, botanical. Here is a closer look at these and other professionals who share the title of "doctor."

Doctors of Medicine (M.D.s)

Medical doctors who are trained in the U.S. have successfully completed an undergraduate degree program after high school (secondary school) that includes at least the required premedical studies covering different course work in biology, chemistry, physics, calculus, and other related studies.

Most of the country's accredited medical schools are able to choose from among the smartest and the highest achieving of the country's undergraduates. Medical school applicants must also aim to score well on a standardized admission test that has been restructured for 2015 to include testing of reasoning and critical thinking skills; knowledge of statistical, social, behavioral, and population sciences as well as cross-cultural awareness; the ability to intelligently and properly interpret research; and a greater variety of skills and scientific competencies across many other disciplines, including information technology.

The next step in medical education is four years of training at an accredited medical school, in accord with established educational standards. Stateside, 141 accredited medical education programs lead to the M.D. degree, with another 17 accredited programs in Canada. For individuals interested in a physician-scientist or academic teaching career track, certain programs offer combined M.D. and Ph.D. training, which requires seven to eight years to complete on average.

Although successful graduation from an accredited medical school program grants the M.D. degree, the vast majority of graduates continue their training by entering a postgraduate or residency program, as generally required for licensure and to be allowed to practice in affiliation with a hospital. The first year of a residency was commonly known as an internship. Depending on the chosen specialty, residency training may last for three to six years after medical school, some of which might be spent doing research. Subspecialty training may require an even longer commitment with fellowship training of one to many years that frequently involves clinical research and the teaching of residents, interns, and medical students.

All in all, medical education entails an additional 11 to 16 years of training after high school—and often more. Medical students begin supervised contact with real patients early in their medical schooling, often during their first year. Students' patient experiences continue to expand in terms of time spent in direct, hands-on care and responsibility as the medical student progresses to his or her fourth year. With internship, the learning curve of a newly minted M.D. soars with regard to in-depth direct patient-care experience and responsibility, increasing in intensity and difficulty with each progressive year.

Throughout medical school, and especially during residency and fellowship training, doctors and doctors-in-training experience thousands of patient encounters. They learn the many ways in which common diseases such as appendicitis or allergies might manifest in different types of people. They encounter rare diseases as well as common diseases that manifest in unusual ways.

Ideally, residents and fellows learn how to reason with an open mind and to avoid pitfalls in diagnosis and treatment, all the while absorbing established knowledge and learning what is new and **evidence-based** and learning which therapies have been shown to be ineffective or harmful.

Teaching students and residents are medical school professors who come from a wide range of disciplines and practice types, presenting a variety of skill sets and points of view, ranging from Nobel Prize winners and internationally known opinion leaders to practitioners who volunteer at free clinics or who tend to the needy at home and abroad.

The settings in which medical doctors learn are also varied and are designed to give trainees broad, specialized, and in-depth experiences. Typically, medical students and residency/fellowship-level doctors rotate through a variety of hospitals and health-care settings such as high-volume, large metropolitan hospitals and trauma centers;

outpatient clinics; military hospitals; psychiatric hospitals or wards; pediatric hospitals; community hospitals and clinics; specialized hospitals or units (for example, HIV, orthopedics, or heart care); rehabilitation facilities; geriatric units; and private hospitals or settings that embrace a different model of care, such as Kaiser Permanente.

The goal during all these years of intensive and wide-ranging experience is to gather an exceptional, practical, and highly diverse learning experience that deepens a doctor's fund of knowledge and that lays a solid foundation for the lifelong learning that is required for continuous professional growth and to maintain skills, competency, and licensure.

Although physician licensure requirements vary from state to state, to qualify as a Diplomate of the National Board of Medical Examiners, a U.S. medical school graduate must, in addition to successfully completing the M.D. degree and (at minimum) 12 months of postgraduate training at an accredited program, show fundamental competence to practice medicine by passing a three-part standardized licensing examination. Almost all practice-bound M.D.s then go on to residency programs that vary in length depending on the specialty.

Is There a Doctor in The House?

When it comes to being called a doctor, it seems as though everybody wants to get into the act, as comedian Jimmy Durante might have joked. Before *Dr. Oz, House,* and *Grey's Anatomy,* television shows have featured fictional and real-life medical doctors since the 1950s. The 1960s brought Drs. Kildare and Ben Casey to homes across America, followed by *Marcus Welby, M.D.,* and the zany doctors of *M*A*S*H* in the 1970s. The sports and entertainment industries churn out other types of "doctors," such as sports legends Dr. J (Julius Erving) and Doc Rivers, the doc musicians (Doc Watson, Dr. Dre, Doc Severinsen), movie characters (Dr. No, Dr. Strangelove), and doctor celebrities, many of whom are instantly recognized by their first names alone. Loquacious, entertaining, and smart as whips, many of the talk show doctors are not medical doctors at all but are rather Ph.D.s, often psychologists.

Can you spot the medical doctor from among these famous doctors? (Find the answer at the end of this chapter.)

1. Dr. Martin Luther King, Jr.
2. Dr. Phil (McGraw)
3. Dr. Ruth (Westheimer)
4. Dr. Norman Vincent Peale
5. Dr. Joyce Brothers
6. Dr. Henry Kissinger
7. Dr. Seuss
8. Dr. Benjamin Spock
9. Dr. Laura (Schlessinger)
10. Dr. Jeffrey S. Bland

Doctors of Osteopathy (D.O.s)

Students who complete a four-year post-baccalaureate doctor of osteopathy educational program achieve the D.O. degree. Along with the training that they receive during schooling, which is very similar to conventional or **allopathic** medical school course work, D.O.s also undergo more than 500 hours of training in manual medicine known as **osteopathic manipulative treatment (OMT)**.

Osteopathic training is greatly influenced by the power of prevention. Osteopathy aims to develop healthy lifestyle habits and to treat the whole person, often using a hands-on approach to physical diagnosis and treatment. Osteopathic care can also include the use of manipulative treatments such as thrust techniques, myofascial release, and others.

Like M.D.s, D.O.s may choose to train and practice in any residency specialty for which they are qualified, including surgery and the surgical subspecialties. Both M.D.s and D.O.s who choose to specialize may be eligible to fulfill the requirements for certification by the corresponding board of the American Board of Medical Specialties (ABMS). Examples of the latter are board-certified orthopedic surgeons or board-certified dermatologists, whether M.D. or D.O.

Interestingly, most osteopaths (65%) practice in settings that are considered the primary care specialties—that is, internal medicine, family practice, pediatrics, and obstetrics and gynecology, which altogether attract only about 25% of medical doctors.

The osteopathic traditions of compassion for patients and community service have led many osteopathic graduates to locate their practices in underserved areas. Despite differences in training and perhaps in outlook, D.O. licensure and scope of practice (what they are allowed to perform within the boundaries of each state's and licensing bodies' laws) are the same as that of M.D.s, as are their medical prescribing privileges.

OMT has been used successfully in a variety of conditions, although some D.O.s do not necessarily use osteopathic manipulative treatments in their practice settings after training. Lower back pain is the most recognized condition that can benefit from OMT, which may not only reduce pain but can also decrease the use of medications and may help avoid surgery. Other conditions besides disorders of muscles and bones that have been shown to benefit from OMT include migraines; menstrual pain; carpal tunnel syndrome; and perhaps certain respiratory disorders, such as pneumonia, asthma, and sinus problems.

The Roots of Osteopathy

According to the osteopathic perspective, the body is capable of summoning inner forces that aid in self-healing. This philosophy was proposed in the late 1800s by Andrew Still, a frontier medical doctor who was aware of limitations in the healing methods of the times, both on the Civil War front and at home, losing three of his children to a meningitis epidemic. Still came to believe that the answer to healing was not in the drugs of that era but that rather in reclaiming health as it related to the body's inner flows and its anatomic alignment or structural relationships.

Still's ideas were not well received at first. He traveled around the Midwest, seeking acceptance of his hands-on approach to healing, which was named *osteopathy* in 1885. Finally established in Kirksville, Missouri, Still's practice grew to the point that he began to train other physicians in his technique and philosophy, eventually establishing the first American School of Osteopathy in 1892. Soon, so many people were traveling to Kirksville to seek care that more railroad lines were needed to serve the region. Although today's practicing osteopaths may not universally accept Still's theories and practices, the osteopathic belief in the healing potential of the body and in physical methods of diagnosis and treatment remain strong.

Source: A.T. Still University Museum of Osteopathic Medicine.[SM]

Since 1980, a new crop of American osteopathic schools has opened, which now total 40 nationwide. These schools produced 5,154 graduates in 2013, or about a quarter of the country's overall medical school graduates—that is, the combined graduates of conventional medical schools and schools of osteopathic medicine.

Certain regions of the country have a higher percentage or total number of osteopaths, such as Pennsylvania, Oklahoma, Michigan (along with much of the Midwest), and Arizona. Even though all osteopaths receive manual manipulative medical training, not all osteopaths continue to use this method in practice. If you are specifically interested in having this care option available to you, be sure to ask a prospective D.O. if he or she incorporates manual medicine into his or her current practice.

Doctors of Pharmacy

When it comes to seeking out a health-care practitioner with different skill sets, pharmacists can provide great value. Yet, although pharmacists are some of the most highly trained and knowledgeable health professionals, they are often overlooked or underappreciated members of the health-care team.

Most pharmacists today have had extensive training in pharmacognosy, the study of drugs made from natural animal or plant material. They also receive highly specialized training in pharmacology, or how drugs of all types act in the body, as well as in toxicology, chemistry, and in the applications of medicines to real-life situations at the bedside, clinic, care facility, or home.

Although pharmacists are generally considered mainstream members of the health-care team, people seeking alternative or integrative care may nonetheless wish to seek their advice. Patient-oriented and wellness-focused pharmacists are emerging as uniquely skilled and important members of health-care teams. These clinical pharmacists help hospitalized patients and outpatients manage and understand chronic conditions such as diabetes, high blood pressure, arthritis, weight control, tobacco cessation, allergies, asthma, severe kidney disease, and Alzheimer's disease.

Unlike some alternative fields of study that have not expanded, adapted, or lengthened to reflect the enormous explosion of knowledge that has occurred across health care, pharmacists are the product of a profession that has tackled those challenges, starting from the fundamental training of would-be pharmacists.

In response to recommendations made by the Institute of Medicine regarding the training and competence of health-care professionals, pharmacy education made a radical change in 2000 when the Accreditation Council of Pharmacy Education put a new set of educational standards into effect. Before that time, most pharmacists were trained as Bachelors of Science in Pharmacy (B.S., Pharm.), a specialized type of bachelor's degree that required five years of study. The new standards scrapped the B.S. in pharmacy degree. In its place, the lengthier and more demanding Doctor of Pharmacy degree was established, which is now the only pharmacy degree available that fulfills the training aspect of licensing requirements, along with demonstrated competence and satisfactory performance on stringent examinations.

Known as the Pharm.D., it requires at least two years of undergraduate study in pre–pharmacy sciences, often as part of an undergraduate degree, followed by another four academic years of professional pharmacy training with thousands of hours of supervised practice in clinical rotations and a six-month externship. Pharmacists seeking advanced practice status or those who wish to work in an academic or hospital pharmacy setting undergo even more training as pharmacy residents or by pursuing related master's or doctoral (Ph.D.) degrees.

Insurance companies and health plans are increasingly recognizing the untapped value of pharmacist-assisted care. Medicare and other health plans offer coverage for certain conditions such as the chronic conditions mentioned earlier and others that involve the participation of pharmacists. Health-care reform may finally help bring these highly trained and hugely resourceful professionals onto the radars of health consumers as well as their professional colleagues. Consider how pharmacists might help you become better informed about natural products.

What Kind of Doctor Is Your Doctor?

Integrative practitioners differ widely in their training level or expertise. Some integrative practices are rooted in formal training, though others are not. Some practitioners are required to demonstrate that they are ethical, adequately trained to perform the services provided, competent, and up-to-date in their field. Again, others are not. When seeking care for your most precious resources—your body, mind, and life itself—it's important to know more about the person sitting on the other side of the couch, desk, prescription pad, or examination table.

Examples of practitioners whose training, knowledge base, and competence are not standardized or recognized by a licensing professional organization of merit are unspecified "nutritionists"; "herbalists"; and a variety of coaches, consultants, and unregulated or self-proclaimed therapists and counselors. While many of these individuals may be providing value, it can be difficult to determine their level of expertise, training and experience. Perhaps more importantly, it can be hard for health consumers—or the practitioners themselves—to assess the boundaries between their knowledge, personal opinions, guesswork, and instinct.

For example, in states that require licensure, licensed massage therapists undergo formal training, obtain credentials, and fulfill the requirements to practice their art as trained professionals. Some may even become certified through organizations such as the National Certification Board of Therapeutic Massage and Bodywork (see the following chapters for more information on the different types of integrative practitioners). In contrast, many self-taught and self-styled individuals may call themselves "nutritionists," an unregulated title.

Here is a look at the training received by and required of certain integrative providers who you may also know as doctors.

Doctors of Chiropractic

Known as D.C.s, doctors of chiropractic undergo training that is different from that of M.D.s and D.O.s. Chiropractors receive their education at one of the country's eighteen chiropractic colleges, perhaps without having completed a formal bachelor's degree. Recognizing such a high degree of variation in chiropractic training, the World Health Organization put forth guidelines for chiropractic education in 2005. Today, although some four-year chiropractic schools require a college degree, 90 hours of college credit suffice for other schools, with a 2.5 minimum grade point average (GPA) out of 4 required for students entering such programs.

Unlike M.D.s and D.O.s, there are no requirements for any length of postgraduate direct patient care residency training after chiropractic school. The types of practice settings that chiropractic trainees experience are far more limited and are less likely to include many **acute** or complex medical or surgical problems compared to M.D. and D.O. training. For example, it is unlikely, if not unthinkable, that a chiropractor-in-training would have in-depth or perhaps any training at all in recognizing or managing some of the life-threatening complications of diabetes, commonly seen in M.D. and D.O. training programs. Yet, many practicing chiropractors view diabetes and other complex diseases about which they may have had limited exposure as within their scope of expertise.

After three years of chiropractic schooling, trainees may serve a one-year clinical experience with a practicing chiropractor, similar to a beginning medical student's clerkship or shadowing. Some may elect to gain experience in a hospital or a veteran's facility, although neither is required.

In all, chiropractors receive more than 500 hours of manual manipulation training, which differs in philosophy, techniques, and applications from that of osteopaths.

To obtain state licensure, chiropractic school graduates take a four-part examination given by the National Board of Chiropractic Examiners, although not all states require passing scores on all four parts. Except in New Mexico, D.C.s are not licensed to prescribe medications and may use acupuncture (if they have successfully completed a brief training program and passed a written exam) and may advise on the use of over-the-counter products.

Despite these differences in their training, experience, and knowledge base, many chiropractors have expanded their practices beyond manipulative and **musculoskeletal** therapies to include their interpretations of care for a wide range of conditions and diseases, including hormonal and immune disorders.

The title of D.C. (doctor of chiropractic) or chiropractic physician is legally permitted for candidates who have successfully fulfilled all licensure requirements. If the abbreviation "Dr." is used before a chiropractor's name—for example, in an advertisement—the practitioner should also specify that he or she is a chiropractor to avoid confusion with a medical doctor.

Doctors of Naturopathy

As a relatively new type of health professional also referred to as "doctor," it can be challenging to understand what type of doctor a naturopathic doctor (N.D.) is and what type of training he or she might have received—and why the answers to these questions matter significantly.

First, not all states regulate and license N.D.s to practice. In addition to five Canadian provinces, the District of Columbia, the U.S. territories of Puerto Rico and the U.S. Virgin Islands, and 17 states in the U.S. offer licensure for N.D.s (Alaska, Arizona, California, Colorado, Connecticut, Hawaii, Idaho, Kansas, Maine, Minnesota, Montana, New Hampshire, North Dakota, Oregon, Utah, Vermont, and Washington). Besides Maryland (scheduled to license N.D.s in 2016), another eight states have legislation pending that would allow N.D.s to be licensed in those states, including many Canadian provinces.

To achieve licensure in those regions where N.D.s are permitted to practice, N.D.s must have graduated from a four-year brick-and-mortar accredited naturopathic program and passed an exam. N.D. degrees conferred by online and correspondence schools are not acceptable for state licensure.

As a result, it can be difficult to know which type of N.D. degree or diploma a practitioner holds because both online and school-based learning grant the same title known as N.D. Perhaps even more confusing for consumers is that the N.D. degree can be called an N.M.D. degree in Arizona (naturopathic medical doctor), according to the practitioner's preferred designation.

The course work of an online or distance N.D. program may require little more than the ability to write legibly, an interest in the subject matter, and the ability to navigate to the payment page. Correspondence students can skip certain courses or may receive advanced credit for "life experience" or other reasons that are not acceptable in accredited schooling.

Moreover, online N.D.s receive little, if any, direct patient-care experience, notwithstanding claims by some of these schools that N.D. students can obtain hands-on experience at the students' homes, with no apparent exclusions for moms or pets. Meaningful clinical supervision by experienced individuals or by scholarly teams in relevant, established practices appears to be absent from these programs. Online N.D. graduates are not eligible to take the standardized exam that is required for state licensure in states where accredited school–graduated N.D.s are permitted.

These types of degree-granting online programs are often able to skirt regulations by claiming religious exemption or by disallowing students from the state where the program is located to enroll in the online study (given that such states do not recognize or regulate the N.D. license granted by the program).

To confuse matters further, in states that do not license N.D.s, graduates of online N.D. programs are nonetheless allowed to use "N.D." after their names, which might mean "naturopathic diploma" rather than "naturopathic doctor." Although these lay naturopaths cannot portray themselves as physicians or attempt to practice medicine, they can associate themselves with and benefit from the expertise that the title "doctor" generally implies to healthcare consumers.

The other type of N.D. has graduated from one of the seven accredited four-year classroom programs at one of the six U.S. naturopathic school campuses (or at the two in Canada) and passed a qualifying exam. Once N.D.s become state-licensed, their scope of practice—that is, the types of care they are legally permitted to render—depends on the state in which they practice. In some states, the N.D. scope of practice is more limited, whereas in states such as Hawaii, Arizona, or Oregon, N.D.s may also be allowed to prescribe certain medications or to perform acupuncture or even minor surgery, typically following a limited amount of additional training or certification.

Health consumers and legislators are often told that naturopathic training is equivalent to that of a medical doctor—an argument that has successfully been used to expand some states' N.D. scope-of-practice laws. This claim is often based on a 2010 study that compared the credits for different subjects in the University of Washington medical school curriculum to those at Washington's Bastyr University's N.D. program during the first two years of basic professional schooling.

Although there was some overlap in the early schoolroom courses in the 2010 Washington study, such course work hardly defines the physician learning experience any more than reading or watching videos about swimming teaches a person how to swim. A meaningful difference in naturopathic compared to conventional medical training regards the far more limited time and resources allotted to diverse patient-care experiences and their comparative lack of supervised hands-on residency training.

Residencies after graduation from naturopathic school are not required and are few in number. Less than 5% of graduates pursue this option, which is where the steepest part of experiential learning occurs for M.D.s and D.O.s. In fact, doctors-in-training in conventional medical programs recognize postgraduate and specialty or fellowship training as providing the most impactful, far-reaching experience and professional skill development.

Utah is the only state to require a 12-month residency for N.D. licensure. In contrast, this is the bare minimum amount of training for the overwhelming majority of M.D.s, previously known as an internship. Outside such training, and perhaps even with it, it can be difficult to reconcile the claims held by many naturopaths that their patient-care experience during lectures and schooling is sufficient to complete and validate their training, to gain adequate and adequately diverse patient-care experience, and to achieve competence on par with that of medical doctors, as claimed in their literature, in promotional materials, and on their websites.

As a health consumer, it is important to understand these differences in health-care provider training among the people who all share the same and powerful title—*doctor*. Ask your doctors what type of doctor they are, where they completed schooling, what type of advanced training they completed and where, what type of license they hold, and whether or not they are certified by a recognized accredited specialty or subspecialty board.

The length and rigor of conventional medical training does not grant M.D.s all knowing or superpowers over other types of providers. Despite such exacting training, knowledge gaps among medical doctors exist. Furthermore, mainstream medical training does not also ensure good people skills, active listening abilities, compassion, or the ability to think beyond conventional care when required.

Medical doctors may express concerns about the limited expertise of other practitioners who are also known as doctors. Such concerns involve the granting of individuals with limited training or more narrow perspectives practice rights that may be at the limits of or beyond their scope of knowledge or experience. Or, as voiced by many conventional practitioners regarding health-care colleagues who may be driving beyond their headlights, they may not know what they do not know.

The Nurse Will See You Now

As with the title of doctor, nurses also reflect a wide range of training, educational level, and skills. Entry-level licensed practical nurses (L.P.N.s, known as licensed vocational nurses or L.V.N.s in California and Texas) work under the supervision of registered nurses (R.N.s) in structured health-care settings. Depending largely on when they completed their training, R.N.s may possess associate- to doctoral-level degrees.

Nurse practitioners (N.P.s) are nurses who have an active R.N. license and who have also had advanced training at a master's, post-master's, or doctoral level from an accredited nurse practitioner program. Their training includes at least 500 hours of supervised clinical training that spans health promotion to pharmacology and physiology, among other advanced disciplines. Some nurses have gone on to doctor of nursing practice (D.N.P.) programs, which offer the highest educational level that nurse practitioners and other advanced practice nurses can achieve. If current trends continue, by the end of this decade the D.N.P. may become the standard entry-level requirement for advanced practice nursing.

As with registered nurses, advanced practice nurse practitioners may also become certified as holistic practitioners. However, a noteworthy difference is that in some states, nurse practitioners are allowed to practice independently—that is, without a doctor's supervision. In 19 states and the District of Columbia, N.P.s may not only treat patients but can also prescribe certain drugs, such as medications to treat high blood pressure and diabetes.

Nurse practitioners are enlarging their footprint on health care. About 350 institutions in the U.S. offer N.P. training, with nearly 200,000 NPs in current practice.

What's more, since 2006 the American Nurses Association has officially recognized holistic nursing as a defined nursing specialty. Learn more about this emerging specialty and how nurse practitioners might satisfy your integrative health-care needs by visiting *aanp.org*.

In later chapters, we'll take a closer look at the training, degrees and certification of integrative practitioners whose practices include therapies such as massage therapy, mind-body practices, acupuncture, and other specialized methods.

WHERE TO LEARN MORE

National Center for Complementary and Integrative Health: *http://nccih.nih.gov*

The National Center for Health Statistics of the Centers for Disease Control and Prevention: *http://www.cdc.gov/nchs/*

American Osteopathic Association: *http://www.osteopathic.org*

American Pharmacists Association: *http://www.pharmacist.com*

American Chiropractic Association: *http://www.acatoday.org*

American Association of Naturopathic Physicians: *http://www.naturopathic.org*

American Holistic Nurses Association: *www.ahna.org*

American Association of Nurse Practitioners: *www.aanp.org*

Academy of Nutrition and Dietetics: *www.eatright.org*

Quiz Answer: 8. Dr. Benjamin Spock was an influential pediatrician who wrote or cowrote more than a dozen books, including the best-selling *Dr. Spock's Baby and Child Care* (1946).

3

Integrative Health: What Consumers Should Know

A S NEWS ABOUT THE LATEST SUPPLEMENT OR A NEW THERAPY CLAMOR FOR YOUR attention, facts about whether or not they work can get lost in the noise of testimonials and advertising. In daily life, we rely on our common sense, knowledge base, and experience to guide us in making other important choices in life. Perhaps we consult a trusted friend or family member. Sometimes, we hit the books or the Internet to find out all we can, as when preparing to buy a new car or deciding whether to refinance a house. Yet, when it comes to figuring out the risks and benefits of health-care–related issues, things can become complicated rapidly. We discover that testimonials may have no bearing at all on what you could experience, whether it comes to dramatic weight loss or relief from chronic neck pain. Even supplement labels themselves offer little guidance or information to help us make better decisions.

Thankfully, the movement toward better-informed decision making in health care that takes stock of evidence, effectiveness, and safety is growing stronger. On many fronts, individuals, groups, and organizations are aiding consumers by taking a closer look at what we know about alternative as well as conventional medical therapies. As a result, certain procedures or treatments that were once widely used or believed to work as intended have been reexamined, revised, or rejected.

A better understanding of our genetic makeup and gene variations has also allowed practitioners to personalize certain treatment approaches. It is hoped that such personalization will help increase the odds that particular methods will work in certain individuals. New genetic discoveries may also help in minimizing the possible risks associated with the use of some treatments for people in whom such therapies are less likely to work. More and more, these concepts are also being applied to integrative health.

Health consumers who are asking questions about what works and what they can expect want and deserve fuller answers. Meanwhile, conventional and integrative practitioners are examining their own assumptions, routines, and decision making to tease out what constitutes best practices and what, if any, evidence exists for the choices made both by practitioners and their patients. The goal is better outcomes overall and the best possible result for each individual seeking care.

NCCIH: Research, Evidence, and Safety

In response to growing consumer and academic interest in CAM, the U.S. National Institutes of Health established the National Center for Complementary and Alternative Medicine (NCCAM) in 1998. What began as an office with $2 million in funding in 1992 has grown to a far-reaching source of funding and research training programs, investigating a wide range of CAM therapies across nine major offices and divisions. The mission of the NCCAM, newly renamed the National Center for Complementary and Integrative Health (NCCIH), is to define the usefulness of integrative therapies and to explore their role in health and health care, all through scientific investigation and research support. Although evidence is held in high regard, the NCCIH site also reports on studies of therapies for which the evidence might be sketchy, inconsistent, or absent. A consumer-friendly website at *www.nccih.nih.gov* provides free and updated information about various studies from investigators across different disciplines, short videos, fact sheets, and an array of helpful consumer tips.

EVIDENCE: THE LONG AND WINDING ROAD

The questions being asked at NCCIH are similar to the questions that are also being applied to mainstream care.

- How does a therapy work?
- Can this effect be studied in people?
- What are the specific effects of the therapy?
- How well does it work in the real world?

The search for evidence begins with basic research that attempts to answer the first question. With an herbal supplement, this might begin with a search for the active ingredients in the herb, and finding out which part of the plant contains that ingredient and in what quantities or strength. Basic research would also examine any potential toxicity of the herb; contamination issues; or its potential for interactions with foods, drugs, or other dietary supplements.

To examine whether or not evidence exists for a given treatment, that therapy must be tested and retested, beginning in the laboratory and eventually in small and then larger groups of people. The research studies involving these test groups are called **clinical trials**.

Once testing and trials have concluded, the results and the design of the studies themselves are further examined. Conclusions that have been drawn by the investigators should be warranted by the actual results, although sometimes these conclusions are overreaching or perhaps too optimistic. A common refrain is that "further studies are needed." Many such trials are performed in relatively healthier individuals, and the results are obtained from small numbers of participants or volunteers. Consequently, the results may look different when that test therapy is applied to the general population, used for a long period of time, or given to people who are much sicker or different than the groups that participated in the experimental trials.

When considering the state of the evidence and the trials upon which evidence is based, these are some of the questions that arise:

1. How well designed were the experiments or trials?
2. Were the tests or the researchers biased or not biased to favor one result or another?
3. Who or what company paid for the study, and could a potential conflict exist?
4. Did the investigators study enough people to detect a result that was real and not just due to chance or something else?
5. Did the trial include an adequate variety of individuals (men, women, different races and ages) upon which to base a recommendation for the general population?
6. Were the test results only obtained from healthy or fit people, and if so, how well can these findings be applied to people who might be less fit or unwell?
7. How accurately were the measurements, data, and findings reported and interpreted?
8. How well have the study findings been reproduced by others?
9. How closely and critically did the investigators explore the potential risks or downsides of the treatment under study?
10. Did the study measure the right things and in the proper way?
11. Was the follow-up period long enough for what was being studied, and did the benefits of the therapy make a difference in the final outcome?

It quickly becomes clear that examining and establishing proof or evidence involving health issues can be a long, expensive, and difficult process.

Notwithstanding these efforts, some practitioners and health consumers are comfortable pursuing treatments for which evidence is incomplete, biased, or unknown. Decisions are often influenced by other factors besides evidence—for example, emotions, individual tolerance for risk, or perhaps the sway of others.

As conflicting headlines show from time to time, evidence gaps exist for many kinds of treatments. Reading or hearing that a therapy that was so highly touted last year has now been shown to be useless, unlikely to help your condition, or, even worse, potentially harmful, is confusing and disheartening for many health consumers. People may become skeptical or distrustful about health news. Some may lose hope of understanding the bottom line as health stories get rewritten and revised following new discoveries or disappointments.

Yet, such inconsistencies are part of the process of discovery. Rethinking methods and practices often indicates that progress is being made. Achieving better health and better health outcomes overall is a slow and evolutionary process. Yet, health progress is often presented to consumers like a series of snapshots, taking form as headlines, new diet books, television blurbs, or a buzz on the Internet that goes viral. In contrast, the process of scientific discovery actually unfolds more like a slow-paced movie. Like a film, health and scientific discovery is backed by a basic story line that is complicated by plot twists, drama, colorful characters, and sometimes, but not always, happy endings. It is through rethinking, remolding, and reexamining that our health knowledge expands. Unlike the instant appeal of snapshot health news, the few monumental improvements in public health that have endured and that have provided profound value for the majority of people have typically been unglamorous and have rarely presented instant rewards. Examples include the establishment of a clean water supply and the use of seat belts.

How Much Evidence Do We Need?

Despite the mountain of scientific knowledge that has been built, we still do not have adequate guidance to make major types of health decisions in certain situations. Acupuncture or pain relievers for neck ache? Heart bypass surgery or major lifestyle changes for heart disease? Chiropractic care or physical therapy for back pain? None of these are simple decisions involving cookie-cutter individuals. Each person and situation will be different and may require different approaches. The dilemma comes in figuring out which approach appears best for that individual.

Notwithstanding the confusion and controversy, certain proofs still emerge and many wrong turns do get righted. For example, evidence is strong that most routine sore throats or colds due to viruses do not need antibiotics. Although it is simple and straightforward, it is a message that still requires repetition and reinforcement. We also know that certain diets once considered healthful, such as low-fat diets, can create another set of problems, especially when less fat means more sugar. With hindsight, this unintended consequence seems crystal clear. However, it took time to appreciate the fallout during and after the low-fat craze.

Having proof or evidence doesn't always lead everyone toward the same, safer path—or that people will follow it at all. Although we have known for decades that cigarette smoking and tobacco use lead to a litany of health problems, including death, one in five Americans still smoke. Worse, perhaps, and despite this knowledge, the use of nicotine-vapor electronic cigarettes is on the rise, especially among youth.

We also know that antibiotics won't help most kids get over an earache any quicker, or perhaps won't be of any use at all, yet parents often demand them. The evidence showing the overwhelming benefits of vaccines is also strong, even though many parents take exception to this and refuse to vaccinate their children from diseases that were once rampant and deadly in the pre-vaccine era.

So is evidence in the eye of the beholder? At times it would seem that way. Health practitioners are not immune either. Practitioners of different stripes and philosophies can cite evidence to support their positions, in direct conflict to the reams of opposing studies offered as evidence by a health professional of a different sway. It's no wonder that health consumers are often confused and befuddled by the noise surrounding health choices and decisions.

PLACEBOS AND PROOF

A placebo is a fake treatment, such as being given a sugar pill instead of a real medicine. Placebos also are used in integrative studies. With sham acupuncture, the needle is placed randomly or not at the established acupoints that acupuncturists would usually target in their treatments. The patient who receives the placebo or sham treatment may think that they are getting the real treatment. Sometimes, this belief alone can help a person feel better or believe that the treatment has worked.

The placebo effect can be very powerful, especially for treatments that involve some type of touch therapy, treatments in which a substance that is taken internally (whether by mouth or another route), or treatments that involve extended contact with a care provider. Estimates of the placebo effect have ranged from 35% to nearly 70% in studies of antidepressant treatments. An effective nonplacebo treatment should show that the desired benefits outpace the effects of the placebo, often by at least twofold.

Another success rate to consider is that of no treatment at all. Many noncancerous conditions are known as self-limited—that is, they will or can be expected to go away on their own. Part of the practitioners' art is in determining who will need treatment and who is experiencing a self-limited malady that may require no treatment beyond minimizing certain symptoms. As with a simple cold, most healthy people will feel better with a "tincture of time" and supportive care alone, unrelated to any treatment or supplement they might have pursued. However, if an individual takes a vitamin, an herb, or a prescription drug and then gets better, they may believe that it was the product or the medicine that made all the difference.

Asking about proof that any given treatment has been shown to work is an important first step in becoming a better health consumer. Be prepared for uncertainty, and keep probing.

Other questions that health consumers may want to consider, look into, and discuss with their practitioners include the following:

- Is there evidence that the therapy being considered works?
- Does the therapy work in people like you with your condition?
- How well does this therapy work compared with other methods?
- What are the risks of the therapy, and how likely are they to occur?
- How safe has the therapy been shown to be in people like you?
- How much experience has there been with the therapy?
- What are the risks of not treating?

Not all conditions and treatments will require the highest level of evidence. For example, the typical kind of back pain that people experience now and then will usually get better within a month or so, regardless of what is done for it. Among treatments or approaches such as rest, massage, over-the-counter pain relievers, physical therapy, chiropractic manipulation, acupuncture, and others, no singular superior treatment has emerged. Here, evidence may give way to preference.

However, with chronic back pain that lasts over time and never really goes away, it becomes more reasonable to investigate the strength of the evidence for chiropractic, massage, supplements, acupuncture, and other types of care, as well as how any of them compare to conventional care. Also important is establishing the safety of any treatment under consideration, including over the long term, and its cost.

SAFETY

When looking into the safety of a CAM therapy, consider these three important concerns.

1. How safe is a particular therapy in general? For example, massage therapy is generally quite safe. Not only are side effects rare, but they also are usually minor in terms of the potential harm they might cause. The benefits far outweigh the risks.
2. How safe is a particular therapy when used by people like you? Using the massage example, a pregnant woman would want to know how safe massage has been shown to be in other pregnant women.
3. How safe is the therapy under consideration compared to another type of CAM therapy and to mainstream medical care?

The pregnant woman in the example above might weigh the safety of massage for her morning sickness versus ginger or acupuncture treatment. Are they all equally safe for a person like her? Also, are these alternatives safer or less safe than other integrative methods or with respect to the conventional options offered by her obstetrician?

Difficult as these questions are to resolve, they are worth examining with your practitioner. Weigh in as an empowered, informed health consumer by engaging your health-care team with your questions or concerns about safety.

On the other hand, many of the decisions we make in life are not guided by safety concerns or even by logic. Not all drivers buckle their seat belts every time. Health decisions, too, are often influenced by preferences, denial, and emotions. This can be especially true for people who live with chronic pain or who have encountered failures or roadblocks with conventional medical care.

For individuals who seek greater wellness or who are interested in self-directed care, trial and error may seem like an acceptable way to experiment with different therapies. However, the playing field may not be equal with regard to safety among different methods, especially for certain health concerns such as diabetes and high blood pressure, conditions for which treatment failure can bring serious consequences.

CAUTION AHEAD: DIETARY SUPPLEMENTS

Safety is especially important for people who take or are interested in taking dietary supplements. Many supplement users take a variety of products daily—perhaps along with their prescription medications and possibly for long periods of time, even years. According to a 2012 survey from the Council for Responsible Nutrition (CRN), a trade association that represents makers of dietary supplements and ingredients, 76% of people who take dietary supplements consider themselves regular users of such products.

Depending on the supplements being taken, such use might be acceptably safe. For the health consumer, however, knowing what is safe, not so safe, or outright unsafe can be tough to figure out.

This uncertainty may not register with many dietary supplement users because most people—a staggering 85%, according to the 2012 CRN survey—are confident in the belief that supplements are safe. The same survey also showed that dietary supplement users felt confident in the quality and effectiveness of supplements.

Similar surveys over the past two decades drew similar conclusions—that is, most Americans consider dietary supplements to be safe, and the majority of Americans believe that they are regulated for quality and have been shown to be effective.

Does this overwhelming show of support match up with the facts? Unfortunately, the answer is no.

The Dietary Supplement Health and Education Act of 1994 (DSHEA)

In the United States, dietary supplements are not regulated as prescription drugs. In fact, even though supplements are taken as self-medication and might possess drug-like actions, supplements are not regulated as drugs at all. Under the Dietary Supplement Health and Education Act of 1994 (DSHEA) that was passed by the U.S. Congress and became federal law, dietary supplements were no longer regulated as food additives but rather were, and still are, considered a category of foods by the Food and Drug Administration (FDA). As a special food category, and with only very limited exceptions, products under DSHEA are not reviewed for safety or effectiveness before they enter the U.S. consumer market and end up in your shopping cart.

What Is a Dietary Supplement?

The DSHEA defined dietary supplements as products (other than tobacco) meant to supplement the diet.

A dietary supplement product may contain any of the following, alone or in combination with other dietary supplements:

- a vitamin
- a mineral
- an herb or botanical
- an amino acid
- a dietary product used to increase dietary intake in humans
- a substance that is found in the diet, such as enzymes
- a related product or constituent of such products, such as concentrates, extracts, organ or gland tissues, metabolites, or a combination of the above

Dietary supplements are also meant to be taken by mouth and are therefore familiar to us in pill, capsule, gelcap, softgel, powder, or liquid forms.

Because dietary supplements occupy a special place in regulatory law, makers of dietary supplements are not required to follow most of the laws, testing, and requirements that apply to prescription drugs.

Also unlike prescription drugs, DSHEA does not oblige manufacturers to list possible risks on their products' labels, even in cases where dietary supplements have been known to have possible side effects or interaction problems, including those with prescription drugs.

These facts often come as a surprise to supplement users. Consumers may believe that because a supplement does not carry a warning label, it is safe to use, even if they are taking other supplement products or prescription drugs. A halo of safety may also encircle products perceived as natural, even when that halo is nonexistent.

Similarly, consumers who have serious underlying conditions such as heart problems, diabetes, or autoimmune diseases such as lupus might mistake the absence of a warning label as an indication that a given supplement is safe in individuals such as themselves who have such conditions.

Sensitive Populations

Whether related to age, development, or special circumstances, certain individuals can be at greater risk of unwanted or unknown effects from dietary supplements or other therapies that are generally safer in healthier or more average-risk people or groups. Below is a partial list of sensitive populations for whom the risks and benefits of any therapy—including those offered by mainstream medical care—should be carefully considered.

- all children and adolescents younger than 18
- older adults
- pregnant women and nursing mothers
- individuals taking multiple medications or supplements
- individuals with multiple medical conditions or chronic diseases
- individuals who are preparing to have surgery or a procedure

Safety, Side Effects, and the Burden of Proof

Not only did the DSHEA exempt thousands of products from evaluation for their safety before Americans were exposed to possible risks associated with their use, but it also shifted the responsibility of proving harmful effects related to these products from the manufacturers (as with prescription drugs) to the FDA and the U.S. government.

Under DSHEA, the FDA and government bodies can act only after a supplement has been made available to consumers and its use has been linked to documented side effects or harm that warrant action. It is the FDA, and not the manufacturer, who must prove that the supplement or certain ingredients in the supplement were clearly linked to the unwanted side effect and that the supplement is unsafe. In the past, these unwanted reactions have included many deaths.

The DSHEA ruling stands in stark contrast to the pre-marketing approval process in place for all prescription drugs. With prescription medicines, the manufacturer must prove that its product is safe and effective according to heavily structured regulations and strict criteria before the drug is eligible for FDA review and approval. Rejections due to safety and efficacy concerns occur frequently.

Even with the extensive studies that are undertaken before a drug even reaches the market, newly approved drugs undergo continued safety testing and surveillance for unwanted side effects after they are out on the market. In this post-marketing period, many more people than were studied in the original experimental trials during the pre-approval phase are now exposed to the new drug. Previously undetected or underappreciated problems can emerge, as with the heart risks that were associated with the prescription drug Vioxx, which led to it being taken off the market.

Because supplement manufacturers are not required to conduct extensive studies of safety, dosages, side effects, interactions with different body systems, and extended use over time in animals and then on to larger groups of human test populations, as they are for prescription drugs, the FDA has needed to take action only after many negative reactions have surfaced. Complicating this situation is the fact that many such reactions to over-the-counter products go unreported.

Dietary Supplement Problems: Flex Your Power

Passed by Congress at the end of 2006, the Dietary Supplement and Nonprescription Drug Consumer Protection Act gives consumers a voice in alerting the FDA to problems with dietary supplement use. Consumers and health-care practitioners can telephone or use an online, fax, or mail-in form to alert the FDA of suspected reactions related to dietary supplements. Adverse events are defined in this case as *any* health event related to a dietary supplement. Serious adverse events are those events that result in hospitalization, a life-threatening experience, death, significant disability, or birth defects, or those that require a medical or surgical procedure to prevent such consequences. Remember that any adverse event, even a seemingly insignificant rash, should be reported.

Supplement makers who receive reports about adverse events are required to report them. Some manufacturers have chosen to ignore such notifications in the past, with deadly consequences. Yet, the manufacturers themselves are often uninformed about problems encountered in the use of their products, highlighting the importance (and shortcomings) of the voluntary reporting system. Supplement makers must complete their own reporting forms. The consumer-friendly **Form FDA 3500** for consumers and health professionals can be found at *www.fda.gov*.

Many of the ingredients used in the estimated 55,000 dietary supplements currently sold in the U.S. have not undergone rigorous safety evaluation. As more Americans choose dietary supplements, more unwanted side effects could be expected to occur. Certain preparations, such as those designed to help build bulk or muscle mass, those designed to improve sexual function, and especially those formulations that are designed to assist in weight loss—often labeled as "fat burners"—have come under scrutiny.

A 2014 study that looked specifically at liver injury due to herbal products or other dietary supplements found that the rate of liver injury in a study group of Americans over a 10-year period increased from 7% to 20%. In this study, the cases with the most severe liver damage involved non-bodybuilding supplements, and most of the severe damage occurred in middle-aged women. These more advanced cases of liver damage more often required liver transplantation and were more often fatal compared to the liver injury cases involving the group taking bodybuilding supplements or to those cases in which the liver injury was associated with conventional medical therapies.

The non-bodybuilding supplements associated with fatal results or the need for a liver transplant in this report included various colonics and cleanse preparations, Ayurvedic products, Chinese herbal mixtures, energy boosters, and an herbal product touted as an alternative to a prescription sexual potency enhancer (*Liver Injuries From Supplements Up 3-Fold in 10 Years in Large Study*. Medscape. Sept. 8, 2014, accessed Sept. 26, 2014).

How Are Dietary Supplements Regulated?

Supplement manufacturers, aiming to counter the bad press that their industry receives with each new wave of supplement scares, FDA warning letters, and movement toward stricter regulation, deny that their industry is unregulated and that their products are potentially unsafe for consumers. Adding to consumer confusion, the website of the NCCIH itself states that the FDA does regulate supplements—noting, however, that the rules for supplements are different and less strict than those for prescription drugs.

Notwithstanding, the answer to the question of whether dietary supplements are approved by the FDA as stated on the FDA website (*www.fda.gov*) is unequivocal: No.

The rules that do apply to dietary supplements primarily involve three aspects: ingredients, manufacturing practices, and labeling.

Regarding ingredients, under DSHEA, supplement ingredients that were sold prior to the 1994 law are considered established ingredients. Such ingredients can be sold without any further proof of safety or effectiveness. However, for any new dietary supplement ingredients introduced after 1994, the FDA requires manufacturers to provide evidence that supports what it calls a "reasonable expectation" of safety.

How well has this largely unenforced ruling fared in practice, and what might this mean for supplement users? Since DSHEA passed in

1994, the number of dietary supplements on the over-the-counter market has grown from 4,000 to more than 55,000, according to 2012 figures. Of the more than 51,000 products that have entered the market since 1994, many would be expected to contain new ingredients.

Although manufacturers are required by law to provide supportive evidence of reasonable safety, according to a 2012 report in the *New England Journal of Medicine*, the FDA had received adequate safety data for only 170 new ingredients used in the more than 51,000 post-DSHEA products being consumed by millions of Americans.

Both the supplement industry and the FDA have recognized the shortfall based on this simple arithmetic regarding ingredient safety reporting. The FDA is exploring new guidance rules for the supplement industry, which in turn has continued to provide feedback to the FDA as this reevaluation process continues toward better consumer safety.

Natural, but Deadly

Nature and what is natural have their ways—some good, some not so good. Rainfall sustains plant life and all that feed on them, while monsoons can ravage terrain and kill living things in its path. Two tragic events involving substances that were considered to be natural products brought increased scrutiny to the dietary supplement market.

In 1989, the amino acid supplement L-tryptophan was associated with an outbreak of a peculiar syndrome that affected more than 1,500 people, causing at least 38 deaths. An investigation into the eosinophilia-myalgia syndrome caused by the L-tryptophan revealed that the supplement maker had altered the purification process to cut costs, a modification that had led to contamination. In 1990, sales of this supplement were banned.

More than a decade later, the FDA banned supplements containing ingredients related to ephedrine after supplements sold as Ephedra caused heart attacks and were linked to serious health effects affecting an estimated 155 people. Among those was a fatal heatstroke reaction in a young major league baseball pitcher. However, a broader investigation revealed in 2007 that the manufacturer had purposefully hidden more than 10,000 health complaints related to their supplements, which were banned by the FDA in 2004.

Another pro-consumer action occurred in 2007 when the FDA required that supplements be made according to current good manufacturing practices, abbreviated cGMPs. Under this rule, manufacturers must follow and document certain practices in the making, packaging, labeling, and storage of supplements. This rule was designed to ensure that supplements contain what they are said to contain on the label and that they are not contaminated by undesirable elements such as impurities, pesticides, or heavy metals.

The cGMP rule, rolled out in phases to allow the supplement industry's smaller and bigger companies to adapt to these new requirements, also requires manufacturers to conform to certain conventions aimed at ensuring that consumers are purchasing the types and amounts of the ingredients that are stated on the label. These rules were also meant to encourage the supplement industry to address the identity of their ingredients—as well as their purity, quality, and strength, which consumers have largely taken for granted or assumed were reliable and consistent, as with prescription drugs.

Confusing these ongoing quality efforts are terms such as "pharmaceutical grade" that are sometimes used with private-label or pricier supplements. However, this term has no regulatory meaning as applied to over-the-counter dietary supplements and can mislead health consumers. In reality, "pharmaceutical grade" refers to compounds or products that have been documented to have been made in accord with strict, established standards of purity and safety that ensure that the product is stable, safe, and effective. Medicines made to those high standards are submitted for FDA approval as prescription drugs, not as dietary supplements.

Although the new cGMP rules were meant to address problems that had occurred in the manufacturing of supplements—including issues with contamination, missing ingredients, or products that contain different amounts than are stated on the label—problems continue to arise.

As one example, in 2013 the FDA removed supplements containing dimethylamylamine (DMAA) from the market after it received nearly 100 reports of sickness, heart attacks, and death related to the supplement ingredient, often touted as a fat burner and a muscle builder. DMAA had been approved in the 1940s as a nasal decongestant, but this approval was rejected in 1983, making the use of this ingredient illegal. Still, DMAA made its way into supplements sold legally in the open market as over-the-counter products. Worsening consumer confusion during the product recall was the fact that DMAA went by at least 10 different names on certain supplement labels, making it difficult for consumers to know if their supplements of choice contained this harmful substance.

Fast Facts About USP Verified

Established in 1820, the US Pharmacopeial Convention (USP) has been setting the definitive quality standards for food chemicals, prescription drugs, compounding, herbals, and supplements for nearly 200 years. The independent nonprofit publishes continuously updated compendia, monographs, and sourcebooks to help manufacturers adhere to strict standards to help guide them in making consistent, standardized products. Although prescription medications must be USP verified, adherence to USP standards is voluntary for dietary supplements under the DSHEA.

An official USP Verified Mark on the label of a supplement assures consumers that it has been carefully tested and evaluated such that 1) the ingredients listed on the label are indeed contained in the product in the stated amounts and in the declared strength; 2) the product does not contain harmful levels of contaminants; 3) the supplement will break down or dissolve and release its ingredients in the body within a certain time period; and 4) the product has been made following current FDA good manufacturing practices using sanitary, well-controlled processes. These procedures include adequate monitoring, quality control, and documentation steps that help to minimize batch-to-batch variations and are intended to heighten attention to quality.

By the same token, it is just as important to understand that the USP Verified Mark does not mean that a dietary supplement is either safe or effective for the condition for which it is being used. In contrast, prescription drugs bearing the USP Verified Mark have been evaluated for safety and efficacy by the FDA.

Source: *www.usp.org*

In another case from late 2014, the FDA ordered a supplement maker in Georgia to stop selling products it was marketing as treatments for different diseases, which are claims that are strictly prohibited under the DSHEA. These supplement products were sold as treatments for diseases ranging from HIV/AIDS to cancer, heart disease, and diabetes, among others. Other cases of dietary supplement fraud have included products that were spiked with prescription drugs or that were diluted or bolstered by inactive fillers such that little or not enough active ingredients remained.

Despite these slow and incremental steps toward greater consumer safety, the FDA website lists hundreds of recalls, warning letters, and other actions it has taken against dangerous ingredients and harmful products in the years since the 2007 cGMP ruling.

The FDA: Consumer Friend or Foe?

Notwithstanding many of the positive steps taken by the FDA to improve consumer choice and to limit the proliferation of potentially harmful or misleading products, many Americans view the FDA, a government agency, with distrust or skepticism.

A national survey of 1,351 adults by a political science research team at the University of Chicago that was investigating the degree to which American adults believed in medical conspiracy theories presented a few surprising statistics in 2014. Among these were that 37% of those surveyed believed that the FDA, under pressure from pharmaceutical companies, is deliberately withholding information about cancer cures and other cures by natural products from the American public. With nearly four in 10 adults subscribing to this belief, this opinion could seem practically mainstream and hardly a fringe belief.

Is the U.S. Leading or Lagging in Supplement Safety?

Stepping away from the FDA, how have other governments or international organizations assessed dietary supplement safety or regulation?

The World Health Organization (WHO) published its first traditional medicine strategy in 2002 regarding native or cultural practices that are distinct from technology-driven mainstream medical care. The document tapped into the expertise not only of the member states but also that of non–United Nation representatives, nongovernmental organizations, and a variety of expert traditional medicine committees and centers.

The WHO report states that despite the growth and diversity in traditional medical practices worldwide, no methods have evolved alongside them to evaluate their safety and efficacy. The WHO especially emphasized problems in evaluating herbal use and dietary supplement use, which are largely untested and are used in populations that are not being monitored for reactions or side effects.

The WHO report specifically states that this unregulated, under-examined use "makes identification of the safest and most effective therapies, and promotion of their rational use more difficult. If TM/CAM [traditional medicine/complementary and alternative medicine] is to be promoted as a source of health care, efforts to promote its rational use, and identification of the safest and most effective therapies will be crucial." (WHO Traditional Medicine Strategy 2002–2005.)

Among the WHO's traditional medicine strategy objectives is the regulation and improved safety profile of herbal medicines. In particular, WHO seeks to bring focus to sustainability, quality assurance, safety monitoring, and emerging knowledge about effectiveness to this important aspect of traditional health care worldwide.

Globally, more and more countries have set regulations regarding dietary supplements. Regulated supplements are the norm in most of Europe; in Scandinavia, Asia, South Asia, Australia, and New Zealand; and across large segments of Africa, the Middle East, and South America. As one example, Germany has classified herbal products as medicinals since 1976. Before they can reach the German market, they must be tested for safety, quality, and efficacy. In the future, perhaps Americans will also benefit from that degree of consumer protection.

Are We Making Progress or Treading Water?

The dietary supplement industry and its political supporters have resisted revisiting or reforming the DSHEA. Senator Orrin Hatch of Utah, home to many large supplement makers and organizations, has been particularly influential.

Pushback has also come from consumer groups and those who equate supplement industry reform with the erosion of consumer choice or from those who underappreciate the uncertainty, safety risks, and fraud issues at work within the supplement world. Several reports from a variety of nongovernmental sources might give such consumers pause.

A 2013 study using a DNA-based method to detect contamination or substitutions in herbal products found that most of the 44 products tested from 12 manufacturers contained DNA fingerprints of plant species that were not listed on the label. One-third of products were contaminated, including substances known to have serious health risks, or contained fillers that were also not listed on the label. Products made by only two of the 12 companies did not have substitute ingredients, fillers, or contaminants.

In a separate 2012 study, a university obstetrician-gynecologist interested in investigating hormone therapy alternatives for his patients tested 36 black cohosh products from online and off-the-shelf retail sources. Similar DNA fingerprinting methods revealed that 25% of the samples were actually a type of nonmedicinal plant from China, and not black cohosh at all.

Supplement fraud is coming under review from other sources as well. In late 2013, *USA Today* published the results of its investigation into consumer fraud and tainted supplements. What the reporters found was that many individuals running the companies that make dietary supplements that were found to be laced with prescription drugs or other undisclosed products had criminal histories or other run-ins with the law, often involving drug and regulatory or fraud crimes. Risky supplement categories in the investigation included those sold for sexual enhancement, bodybuilding, and weight loss.

It is difficult to imagine the firestorm that would ensue if it were found that one-quarter of antibiotics were actually inactive or inert, or that most of the blood pressure medications on the market contained other undisclosed drugs or potentially dangerous contaminants. It is worth taking stock of the regulatory gaps and safety issues discussed here—known and unknown—when considering dietary supplementation, especially in at-risk individuals, over the long term, or in combination with other products or medicines.

BECOMING A BETTER HEALTH CONSUMER

Consumer choice continues to grow at an explosive rate. The Internet, social media, and economic booms in various corners of the world have brought even greater choices in integrative treatments and dietary supplements. As recurring episodes and tragedies have shown, many of these choices may be untested or unsafe and bear no guarantee that they will work for what ails us or fulfill the expectations we may hold.

With all the available options to pursue clean and current good manufacturing practices, why, you might ask, don't more supplement companies aim to make better, more purified, and consistent products? Among the many possible answers are that 1) dietary supplement purchases are heavily influenced by price; 2) following these rigorous standards is expensive as well as equipment- and labor-intensive; and 3) manufacturers are not required or incentivized to do so.

As with the polypharmacy that occurs with prescription drugs— that is, the taking of multiple prescription medicines—polyherbacy, or the taking of many herbal products or dietary supplements, is on the rise. So are the expectations of problems and interactions.

The new DNA fingerprinting method is helping scientists determine the amounts, identity, and quality of dietary supplement ingredients. Using sophisticated DNA barcoding techniques, scientists are learning the distinctive DNA signatures that can be used to detect contamination, purity, or substitutions in herbal products. Further progress using this technology or stricter regulatory actions that ensure quality control from seed to shelf are bound to help guide consumer choice toward safer, cleaner product purchases.

Over time, as the better-standardized products of the future undergo testing in human trials, we will learn more about what really does work, at what dose, and for what conditions. By using more consistent products, we will also understand these products' safety profiles, both alone and in combination with other medicines or natural products. Evidence of their effectiveness or lack thereof will be strengthened.

That day may be a long time coming. In the meantime, consider these steps when making choices among dietary supplements:

- Discuss your medication and supplement use with all your providers —including all the dietary supplements you are taking, such as vitamins.
- Review the label for any ingredients you may be allergic to or that might cause problems, including hormones, unfamiliar ingredients, long lists of ingredients, or ingredients that may cause problems such as a rise in blood pressure or heart rate.
- Look for the USP Verified Mark on vitamins and supplements.
- Consult with a hospital-based, clinic-based, or retail pharmacist about different supplement choices and possible interactions with prescription drugs, foods, or other supplements.
- Only buy as much as you are likely to consume before the expiration date.
- Question polypharmacy and polyherbacy—aim to simplify your medication regimen in consultation with your health-care providers.
- Avoid supplements that advertise miracle cures or immediate results and that promise to help you achieve something you know to be difficult, such as weight loss, super strength, a headful of hair, or regained youth.
- Remember that dietary supplements cannot be sold or advertised to cure or alleviate a disease—if they promise to do so, be especially suspicious.
- Certification by an independent laboratory may be as reliable as no certification at all with respect to the specific bottle sitting in your medicine cabinet—look for supplements that follow established, tested procedures, such as those bearing the USP Verified Mark.
- Follow the label instructions—whether a product claims to be natural or not, more is not necessarily better, and more could be harmful.

WHERE TO LEARN MORE

Before you try a new supplement, read about its uses, safety, and the evidence to date from a reliable website such as the free dietary supplement fact sheets from the Office of Dietary Supplements (*http://ods.od.nih.gov*), the NCCIH (*www.nccih.nih.gov*), Medline Plus (*http://www.nlm.nih.gov/medlineplus/druginformation.html*), and the product monographs from Health Canada (*www.hc-sc.gc.ca*).

Helpful information is also available from for-profit websites such as ConsumerLab (*www.consumerlab.com*) or LabDoor (*www.labdoor. com*; paid subscriptions are required for detailed access), which also provide details about specific brands.

A consumer version of the Natural Medicines Comprehensive Database is available as a paid subscription at *www.naturaldatabase.com*.

Among their efforts in developing international standards in the terminology and classification of the world's traditional health systems, the World Health Organization provides publications and information on medicinal plants and traditional medicine as practiced in different parts of the world, including the South-East Asia and Western Pacific regions: *http://www.who.int/topics/traditional_medicine/en/*.

The European Medicines Agency provides a wealth of information about natural and herbal products, including specific herbal monographs at *www.ema.europa.eu*.

4

Integrative Health and You

A S EXPLORED IN GREATER DEPTH IN THE FOLLOWING CHAPTERS, INTEGRATIVE practices vary widely in their use, nature, adaptability, acceptance, reliability, effectiveness, and safety—and the list goes on. Because of these differences, understand that what might be said about massage or acupuncture might not necessarily apply to biofeedback, meditation, or Reiki.

Similarly, the skills, training, and types of practitioners you are likely to find within each integrative field are also quite variable, from highly trained and certified licensed acupuncturists to self-taught herbalists and color therapists or practitioners with many years of rigorous and broad-based training.

Because of these striking differences and the huge number of choices among integrative techniques and therapies, deciding which integrative methods may best suit your overall health plan can be a challenge. Here, we take a look at where you might begin.

IS INTEGRATIVE CARE RIGHT FOR YOU?

Start first by taking stock of your needs and goals. Framing these needs and goals are other factors such as your age, your own personal and family health history, your social and cultural norms, and your lifestyle considerations. Also important are your own beliefs about health, control, and fate, and your ability to adapt to change or to tolerate uncertainty. Faith may also play an important role in choosing the road to health that best accommodates your beliefs and persona.

On a more secular level, the type of work you do and the type of employer you have can also affect your choice of health practices and practitioners. For example, if you have a demanding job with set hours and few chiropractors in your community with office hours that would accommodate your schedule, you may not be able to

49

pursue a chiropractic treatment that requires once-weekly visits for a couple of months.

Finances also matter, as does your insurance status. Because only a limited, although growing, number of integrative treatments are covered by most insurance policies, you will need to consider what and how many treatments are covered along with how well you can absorb additional out-of-pocket expenses and for how long.

Conventional Care: Hits and Misses

When sudden or new health situations arise, such as a cut that needs stitches, being involved in an auto accident, or an abnormal pain that signals the need for immediate help, Western medicine is usually up to the task. Even though the outcomes are not always ideal, conventional care tends to perform well for people with acute illnesses and injuries.

Conventional care also delivers life-changing results in a variety of nonemergency situations, from restoring sight through highly technical and delicate cataract surgery to replacing a worn-out hip with a durable prosthesis that restores mobility and eliminates pain.

Yet, when it comes to chronic illnesses and conditions such as chronic pain syndromes, allergies, diabetes, weight concerns, arthritis, and many others, conventional care often comes up short. Besides not having all the necessary tools and treatments to help relieve or cure chronic conditions, the health-care system itself doesn't step up its game for chronic care to the extent that it does in the acute setting.

Chronic conditions from Alzheimer's disease to cancer are complex and not easy to fix. Altogether, chronic conditions are the most common, costly, and preventable of all health problems, affecting at least half of all American adults.

Reasons to Consider Integrative Methods

People who are affected by chronic conditions that affect their quality of life, often on a daily basis, frequently consider integrative methods. Some may reject conventional care outright, especially if they have had bad experiences with doctors, hospitals, or other care settings. Others may have reached a plateau or are no longer benefiting from the therapies that mainstream Western medicine offers. Some may have been disappointed by the limitations of a treatment, its failures, or burdensome side effects.

For many of these individuals, integrative care may offer a way to gain better control over healing. It can also encourage its users to maintain optimism and hope about future wellness. For many CAM users, choosing such therapies provides a way to grow, both physically and spiritually.

People who use integrative methods may also develop satisfying, healing relationships with their providers, especially since many integrative practitioners tend to spend more time with their clients and patients and personally engage with them more. Patients may find this friendly, collaborative approach to care a welcome contrast to the passive, impersonal, or paternalistic type of care often experienced during rushed or robotic visits in conventional health systems.

Seeking out CAM can also reflect a desire or a need for more personalized attention. CAM users often mention their desire to be heard—to have a practitioner who listens actively and without judgment, insensitivity, or haste. Such individuals might also prefer a health-care provider who spends more time with them—or merely someone who is better able to convey more care, interest, and compassion.

People who use integrative methods also voice a desire to focus on what conventional medicine sees as subjective issues—that is, how individuals feel; what their pain or discomfort is like; and what the effects of their illness are on their quality of life or on other aspects of their emotional, social, and interpersonal lives.

When people decide to follow their own health guidance in choosing integrative methods, their engagement in something other than conventional medicine isn't colored by the passive, out-of-control feelings that are common in mainstream settings. Rather, the pursuit of other types of care may be infused with energy, optimism, and a can-do feeling. Integrative care is also less likely to cause feelings of helplessness or the impotence and frustration associated with being bounced around from referral to referral, drug to drug, or clinic to clinic.

Because many CAM providers are skilled listeners who appear to appreciate more greatly the value of a satisfied customer—you—experiences with integrative providers may radiate greater hopefulness and more satisfying interactions.

On the other hand, people who have been used to or who have had success with many of Western medicine's quick fixes can feel impatient with certain CAM therapies. For example, a person with arthritis may need to take the dietary supplement glucosamine for many weeks before they feel any differently, if at all.

Alternatively, self-guided individuals and people who actively seek out integrative care may derive some degree of relief from a chronic condition that is in part driven by the fact that they are acting as in-control decision makers. As such, they may feel empowered about doing something positive to aid their health and well-being.

SPEAKING UP ABOUT INTEGRATIVE CARE

Regardless of the reasons or expectations for seeking out CAM, at least two out of three people simply do not share this information with their conventional medical practitioners. In a survey of older Americans, the most frequent reason given for not disclosing the use of CAM was that the health-care provider did not ask (42%, 2006 and 2010 data). Another 30% of people surveyed stated that they didn't think that they had to tell their doctor or health-care provider. Almost another 20% felt that there was not enough time to talk about it or that the provider didn't know about the topic. Fewer people were not comfortable discussing CAM, and fewer still either saw no reason to disclose the information (4%) or didn't believe in CAM (3%).

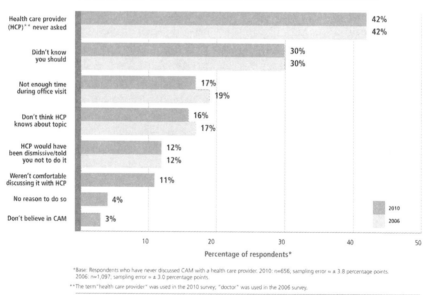

Reasons CAM Was Not Discussed With Health Care Provider

*Base: Respondents who have never discussed CAM with a health care provider. 2010: n=656; sampling error = ± 3.8 percentage points. 2006: n=1,097; sampling error = ± 3.0 percentage points.

**The term "health care provider" was used in the 2010 survey; "doctor" was used in the 2006 survey.

Source: AARP/NCCAM Survey of U.S. Adults 50+, 2010.
Credit: National Center for Complementary and Integrative Health, NIH, DHHS.

What these and other similar surveys of different population groups tell us is that doctors, other conventional practitioners, and patients can all do a much better job of disclosing and discussing this vitally important information.

When health professionals take a detailed medical history and ask what can seem like endless questions about past illnesses, they are trying to develop as complete a picture as possible about a person's health. Complete that picture for all members of your health-care team by speaking openly about your interests in, use of, or desire for integrative care.

More Reasons to Discuss CAM with Your Provider

Providing information about all the treatments and therapies you may be pursuing is vitally important information, regardless of whether or not the practitioner receiving this knows much about them or even agrees with such pursuits. This openness is especially important when it comes to dietary supplements, even seemingly harmless ones such as multivitamins.

For example, people who take thyroid replacement for the fairly common condition of hypothyroidism are advised not to take vitamins, antacids or supplements that might contain iron or calcium within four hours of taking their thyroid replacement medication. Even high-fiber diets or caffeine might interfere with absorption of this vitally important hormone. By not informing your care team that you routinely take your thyroid replacement plus a vitamin with your morning coffee, the reason why your thyroid medicine doesn't seem to be working well enough at what seems like a correct dose may be obscured or go undetected.

Other more serious examples abound, especially with regard to certain herbal supplements or certain conditions that require specialized medications, such as therapy for HIV, cancer, blood clotting disorders, and especially liver and kidney conditions. Being truthful and thorough about any supplements you may be taking is particularly important in older adults, children, pregnancy, and cancer care (including survivorship), and for people with complex conditions or who are taking multiple medications and/or multiple supplements.

Meeting Resistance: What to Know, What to Do

Because conventional practitioners can be skeptical or uninformed about integrative care, or may disapprove of different types of supplements or therapies, many people withhold information or decide it's not worth bringing up. However, you can take a proactive approach toward informing your providers about the choices you've elected to make.

Envision "the talk" as another milestone toward taking greater control over your health. These discussions can also foster better communication and perhaps a more satisfying partnership between you and your doctor toward better health.

How, you might wonder, can anyone be expected to accomplish this, especially when office visits are brief, are often rushed, or occur at times when the provider is not in a receptive or accepting frame of mind?

Fortunately, you can use one or many of the following strategies to introduce and discuss CAM or your desire for an integrative care plan with your provider:

1. **Come prepared.** Make a list of all the over-the-counter supplements and medications you are taking. Include specifics about the dose, brand, and how often you take them (with meals, at night, only when you feel you should take one, etc.). To simplify matters, put the supplement bottles in a bag that you can bring with you to the office or clinic visit. Save precious visit time by making a list that will also provide you with a record that you can keep for your own reference. Your list will also come in handy for relatives, live-ins, or caregivers should they need to access that information in an emergency.

2. **Inform an assistant.** If your provider works with a nurse, nurse practitioner, physician assistant, or another office colleague with whom you feel comfortable, discuss your interest in or use of CAM with that person. Some of these practice extenders should be able to record your history in your chart or to introduce the topic to the primary provider if that is something that makes you feel uncomfortable or hesitant to do on your own. As the chart below shows, you are not alone. Remember, too, that you can bring up CAM to your pharmacist, especially in the special situations of cancer care, multiple medications, and other complicating circumstances, as described earlier.

3. **Get it into your record.** When you are filling out the history forms in the office or prior to your visit, include your other therapies and/or the supplements that you use, including any vitamins, diet aids, custom herb blends, or other nutritionals.

4. **Be proactive.** Don't wait for your doctor to bring up CAM or to ask you about it. Integrative care may not be on your doctor's radar that day—or ever—but if it's on your radar or if it's important to your health vision, make sure to give CAM the emphasis it deserves with regard to your care plan.

5. **Get your questions or declarations in early.** Don't be shy about introducing your feelings, questions, or experience with CAM at the beginning of the visit, especially when the doctor asks about what has brought you in that day or how you are

doing. One way to mention CAM is to answer the question about how you are feeling and then to immediately add, for example, "Before I forget, I want to make sure that you saw that I've been taking selenium lately." Once you make a simple declaration at the start of the visit, you can inform your doctor of any other therapies that you are following so that the practitioner can frame, or reframe as needed, your care plan with you that day and make any necessary adjustments to your medications, treatment, or follow-up schedule.

Types of Health-Care Providers CAM Is Discussed With**

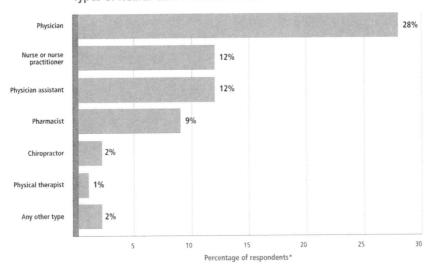

*Base: All respondents (n=1,013). Sampling error: ±3.1 percentage points. Respondents could choose more than one answer.
**All respondents were asked if they had discussed CAM with each type of practitioner; only "yes" responses are shown ("no" and "don't know/no response" are excluded).
Source: AARP/NCCAM Survey of U.S. Adults 50+, 2010.
Credit: National Center for Complementary and Integrative Health, NIH, DHHS.

6. **Don't miss the boat.** Try not to leave "the CAM talk" for the end of the visit, as the doctor is heading out the door. Doing so is counterproductive for a couple of reasons. First, the doctor might be surprised or annoyed about entering into another round of questions and inquiry. Perhaps the doctor will bristle at having to revise all or part of what has already been discussed, planned, or explained to you. Second, doctors who hold strong, uninformed, or negative opinions of CAM are not likely to receive such information or requests at the end of the visit as welcome news or as the best time to open up

communication. Avoid putting the practitioner on the ropes or feeling unprepared to address your health issues by not leaving such an important topic for the end of the visit.

7. **Once the topic has been introduced, start asking questions.** Now that your doctor is better informed about your use of or interest in CAM, begin asking what opinion or suggestions he or she can offer. Most doctors will be up front about what they know or don't know—and most will offer an opinion if you allow them to do so. Even if your practitioner doesn't have direct experience with the CAM method you've chosen or are curious about, he or she may nevertheless know a lot or a little about it. Doctors and other health professionals tap into a variety of health information channels daily (and most nights, too), whether by reading medical journals, reviewing safety alerts and medical newsletters, attending conferences, looking into recent media exposure of a hot health topic, having discussions with other colleagues, engaging in continuing education, or other means. Start the conversation. Ask your provider to look into it further if he or she has a knowledge or experience gap—both of you might end up surprised or enlightened by the results.

8. **Keep learning and sharing.** If you are new to CAM or are sharing with your doctor your desire to look into a different approach for your condition or wellness, keep the lines of communication open. Update your care team about your integrative experiences. Doctors enjoy learning from their patients—it is, after all, an essential part of growing as a medical professional, no matter the specialty, years of practice, or the initials after a practitioner's name. For example, if you have had great success with a chiropractor you've seen for back pain, let your doctor know. Your M.D. may want to know about or to get to know other chiropractors in the community to recommend to other patients in the future.

HOW TO ADDRESS CONFLICT WITH YOUR HEALTH PROVIDER ABOUT CAM

OK, you've done it. You've informed your doctor about your CAM choice or desire for integrative care—but he or she is not happy. Perhaps your doctor has expressed outrage, disappointment, scorn, or feelings of betrayal, or has even poked fun at your choice. Now what?

First, as hard as it may be, attempt to stay on an even keel and to avoid defensiveness. Hear out your practitioner's concerns. Some or all of them could be valid or based on knowledge you hadn't imagined your doctor possessed. Listen actively to what your provider is saying rather than concentrating on your rebuttal or point. Insist that he or she do the same for you.

If you suspect the topic might be a lost cause or more trouble than it is worth, a good way to end the conversation on a less electrified note could be to say, "Thank you for letting me know. I'll keep your concerns in mind" or "I appreciate your frankness. I'll keep you posted."

You can also gently remind your doctor that your integrative choice or interest means a lot to you by merely stating that in a matter-of-fact way. Then, invite him or her to offer help. One way to do this is to say, for example, "This is an important decision for me, and I'd like your help and support."

If you wish to register your unhappiness with your doctor's response without further inflaming the situation, especially if you hope to continue your care with that provider, consider closing the discussion at that time with the response, "I had hoped for a different response. I appreciate your concerns and will keep them in mind. Thank you."

Doctors don't enjoy difficult conversations any more than non-physicians do. Think about what your doctor expresses to you. Chances are good that the doctor is doing the same. If you stay focused, acknowledge what's been said (without having to necessarily agree or argue points), and have attempted to keep the doors of communication open, your chances of maintaining your relationship and reintroducing or reevaluating the subject at a later time will be improved.

Trouble Ahead? Special Considerations

One reason why many Western practitioners may not embrace integrative health, or at least some aspects of CAM, is because of a few uncertain or risky areas involving CAM in their field of practice, whether real or perceived. Although you probably looked up a great deal of information about your choice of therapy or practitioner, keep an open mind about what your mainstream provider has to say when he or she expresses concern about safety or another aspect of integrative care. Your provider may be aware of something that you have not fully considered or that may have merit.

An example is the use of **antioxidants** in cancer care, which is discussed more fully in Chapter 11. By protecting the body against the harmful effects of known or potentially harmful, oxidized substances, antioxidants can be effective disease fighters and prevention agents. Well-known and popular antioxidants include vitamins such as C and E, lutein, and the vitamin-A precursor beta-carotene; lycopene (found in tomatoes); and selenium, among others.

Although zapping harmful **free radicals** by eating antioxidant-rich foods or perhaps giving yourself an antioxidant boost by using supplements could sound like a win-win situation, a downside may exist for certain people. For cancer patients, whether they are actively undergoing treatment or enjoying survivorship, certain supplemental antioxidants may be a double-edged sword. This is because antioxidants are not only able to protect normal cells, but they may also safeguard premalignant or cancer cells from certain anticancer therapies.

Studies have shown that the antioxidants Vitamin E and N-acetylcysteine (sold over the counter as NAC) can actually increase the cancer burden and the death rate in an animal model. These experiments have shown that while antioxidants consumed in the diet do indeed dial down the harmful effects of certain molecules such as reactive oxygen species (ROS) throughout the body, cancer cells have developed their own game plan to combat ROS. These adaptations have allowed cancer cells to, in effect, hijack ROS, using ROS instead to further even greater malignant cell growth. Meanwhile, cancer cells can adapt by repairing the damage caused by ROS on certain molecules in the cancer microenvironment that would have spelled doom for the cancer cells had the antioxidant not been present.

This recent finding might help to explain why many studies that have followed human patients have not been able to show that antioxidants consumed in the diet actually decreased the number of cancers that arose over a period of time, a measurement known in the scientific literature as the incidence. Instead, in the case of men who smoked and who were therefore at risk for lung cancer, there is evidence that some antioxidants (in this case, Vitamin E and beta-carotene) have actually been associated with higher rates of cancer development.

Similar, perhaps even stronger concerns about the use of antioxidant supplements exist for cancer patients who are undergoing treatment with radiation. Notwithstanding, it is important to note that although the evidence against certain antioxidant supplements during cancer therapy has strengthened in the past few years, controversy remains. Most health practitioners agree that there is no need to ban antioxidant-rich foods from the diets of cancer patients and survivors. Rather, good nutrition is always important, and anti-oxidant-rich foods supply many other health benefits and nutrients. Antioxidant supplements, or certain ones in particular situations, may be a different matter.

Understand that conventional medical doctors and alternative practitioners have weighed in on both sides of this argument. Many integrative oncologists support the use of certain antioxidants during cancer care. Talk out this important topic with your health-care team to determine the best choice for you.

Besides antioxidants, certain dietary supplements can interfere with many of the drugs used during cancer care or may cause unneeded stress on key organs such as the liver. Among these are St. John's wort, garlic extract, echinacea, and—especially with regard to the liver—kava kava.

However, as discussed later on, many nutrients, botanicals, and dietary supplements may be useful in cancer care, providing another good reason to fully disclose and discuss your care plan with all of your treating physicians and providers.

Autoimmune disorders include a variety of conditions that also demand special consideration when using CAM. These disorders include the inflammatory types of arthritis such as rheumatoid arthritis. Some of the better-known autoimmune diseases are Sjögren's syndrome, Type 1 diabetes, multiple sclerosis, psoriasis, lupus, vitiligo, Graves' disease, and certain other types of thyroid disease.

Because many supplemental nutrients and products affect the immune system or might have toxic or medication-interfering effects in individuals who have autoimmune disease, be sure to discuss all the supplements that you take with your health-care provider. As discussed in other sections of this book, a number of integrative treatments appear to be beneficial in autoimmune disorders. Speak with your provider about finding the optimal, safest therapies.

Two very important groups of individuals who warrant special consideration when it comes to CAM are children and pregnant women. While the reasons for this might seem obvious to some, it's worth emphasizing that these two groups have special needs when it comes to all types of intake, from getting enough protein and nutrients to requiring special protection from substances that might hinder growth and development, be they ultraviolet radiation from sunlight or lead and other metals. If you are pregnant, considering pregnancy, or considering the use of CAM therapy for your children—especially supplements—be sure to keep your practitioners informed.

At the other end of the spectrum, **older adults** also warrant special consideration when it comes to CAM—again, mostly with regard to supplements. While many older adults are in good health or may take no or very few medications, the use of multiple medications is increasingly common as we age. Such polypharmacy or multiple medication use is also growing among the youth population, many of whom are now burdened by diseases that we traditionally had associated with advancing age, such as high blood pressure, diabetes, high cholesterol, arthritis, obesity, and metabolic syndrome, among other conditions.

More than a third of older adults take five or more prescription medications daily. Besides the potential for interactions among prescription drugs, the addition of over-the-counter supplements may further complicate or possibly pose hazards to an individual's health. Have a full and updated list of all the medicines and supplements you take on hand when you visit your practitioner, and be sure to troubleshoot (and hopefully simplify) your medication list at every visit. A consultation with a pharmacist can also be helpful to better coordinate or simplify your care plan.

HIV is another special consideration with CAM. Care for people who have HIV, the human immunodeficiency virus that causes AIDS, remains complex. A 2014 study reported that persons living with HIV took between six and eleven different medications per day. Since many dietary supplements are known to interfere with antiretrovirals and other medicines commonly used in HIV care (with even more supplements that are either suspected of interfering or that haven't been adequately investigated for potential problems), discussing CAM therapies with your practitioners takes on special importance.

Take the important step toward better communication with your health-care provider and a more complete vision of health by bringing up CAM to all of your providers. In most cases, such discussions can foster learning and acceptance in both directions along your path to holistic healing and health.

WHERE TO LEARN MORE

Office of Cancer Complementary and Alternative Medicine (OCCAM): *http://cam.cancer.gov/cam/*

Talking about Complementary and Alternative Medicine with Health-Care Providers: A Workbook and Tips from the OCCAM: *http://cam.cancer.gov/cam/talking_about_cam.html*

"Time to Talk" information for patients, NCCIH: *https://nccih.nih.gov/timetotalk/forpatients.htm*

5

Integrative Methods and Their Uses

W HETHER YOU'RE NEW TO INTEGRATIVE MEDICINE, CURIOUS ABOUT IT, OR are already a dedicated user of one or more CAM methods, choosing from among the variety and number of different therapies can seem daunting.

To familiarize yourself with which integrative methods are being used in the U.S. by 34% of adults and for what reasons, let's look at the most common reasons given by people for pursuing CAM to understand how far-ranging their health conditions can be.[1]

Among U.S. adults, back pain is the number-one condition for which CAM is used, cited by nearly one in five CAM users. The next most frequent are neck and joint pain, followed by arthritis and anxiety. Rounding out the rest of the top 10 reasons people use CAM are for cholesterol, head and chest colds, other types of musculoskeletal conditions (that is, afflictions of the bones, joints, muscles, and connective tissues such as fascia, ligaments, and tendons), severe headaches or migraines, and insomnia.

While many more reasons exist for using CAM, taking stock of the top reasons reveals that most of these conditions are first, **chronic**— that is, conditions that are present or linger over the course of many weeks, months or years, whether due to a sudden cause or not—and second, most involve pain of some kind. Chronic pain typically does not improve significantly over time.

Because the conditions for which people seek out CAM primarily involve chronic conditions as well as pain, and because chronic diseases are typically resistant to complete cure, their treatment may also be long term, whether through CAM or conventional medicine. As with any mainstream medical therapy that extends over a long period of time, safety must also be the watchword with integrative therapies.

---

[1]Data source: Barnes PM, Bloom B, Nahin R. CDC National Health Statistics Reports #12. *Complementary and Alternative Medicine Use Among Adults and Children: United States, 2007.* December 2008.

WHAT TYPES OF INTEGRATIVE CARE DO PEOPLE USE?

According to the CDC National Health Statistics in 2007 and 2012 update that assessed CAM use by American adults, dietary supplements or natural products lead the list. Natural products were the top choice, with nearly one in five American adults choosing nonvitamin and nonmineral supplements, followed closely by deep breathing, yoga (along with tai chi and qi gong), chiropractic or osteopathic manipulation, and meditation. The next most popular methods included massage, diet-based therapies, homeopathy, progressive relaxation, guided imagery, acupuncture, energy healing, naturopathy, hypnosis, biofeedback, and Ayurveda.

Children have far fewer chronic conditions than adults. Although they do not use CAM as much as adults, the 2012 national health statistics report showed that CAM is being used in kids for many of the same conditions and a few different ones, as shown below:

Conditions Associated with CAM Use Among U.S. Children	Percentage (whole number)
Back/neck pain	9%
Chest or head cold	5%
Anxiety/stress	3%
Other musculoskeletal condition	6%
Attention deficit-hyperactivity disorder (ADHD)	2%
Insomnia	2%

As might be expected, the types of therapies used in children are different from the most frequently used methods among adults. For example, natural products are most popular, followed by chiropractic or osteopathic care, yoga (along with tai chi and qi gong), deep breathing, and homeopathy, with much of the latter appearing to be self-care–directed and less often related to the care of a homeopath. Rounding out the top 10 most popular methods in kids were meditation, special diets, massage, guided imagery, and movement therapies.

Supplement use was also different among children. As with adults, fish oil took the lead among nonvitamin, nonmineral products (used by 1% of children in the recent 2012 health statistics survey), whereas among kids, this was followed by melatonin, probiotics/prebiotics, and echinacea.

Although other surveys show some variations in these statistics, a few themes emerge. Among the most important are:

- The use of integrative methods is on the rise.
- Many different types of therapies are being used.

- Chronic conditions account for a large percentage of CAM use.
- Symptom relief and pain relief are two of the most important conditions for which people seek out CAM.
- Disease prevention and wellness are important drivers of CAM.

As the last point illustrates, integrative methods are being used not only to obtain relief from symptoms or pain but also to enhance well-being, pursue wellness, and perhaps to prevent certain diseases or conditions. For instance, people at risk for or who already have a heart condition may be interested in exploring integrative therapies such as meditation or herbal supplements—for example, red yeast rice (which has been shown to lower cholesterol), fish oil, or coenzyme Q10 (CoQ10, an antioxidant) to help maintain heart health with the aim of preventing more serious heart problems down the line.

Cancer survivors are also attracted to CAM therapies in hopes of preserving or boosting their immune function and their internal defenses. They may see integrative methods as providing a path that is in harmony with their efforts to live healthier and as a way to bolster their bodies' ability to fend off a cancer recurrence.

Many healthy people and older adults also turn to CAM in their quest to stay as healthy as possible for as long as possible. Beyond exercising and watching their diets, healthy individuals may also participate in yoga for health and wellness or seek out other therapies ranging from naturopathy to dietary supplements to regular chiropractic care.

With such a wide range of goals driving the use of so many different kinds of CAM therapies, it can be difficult to size up which therapies are completely safe, somewhat safe, somewhat risky, or potentially harmful for any given condition. To complicate matters further, it can require effort to find a reliable and unbiased opinion regarding the safety of a given therapy for your specific health situation.

Riding alongside safety concerns are questions of effectiveness, sometimes called efficacy. Simply stated, efficacy relates to whether or not a therapy works. Health consumers will also want to know if a certain treatment has been shown to work in people who have conditions similar to the one for which they are contemplating or pursuing that treatment. As one example, if you are a woman experiencing sleeplessness or a new sleep disorder that began once you hit menopause, you will want to know whether the integrative method you are considering has been shown to work in women like you.

Another important question for prospective or active CAM users is whether one type of therapy seems to work better or worse than another therapy for a given individual and his or her condition, known as comparative effectiveness. For instance, should a middle-aged man with back pain expect to get the same degree of relief from chiropractic care as from acupuncture? Likewise, how would conservative conventional medical care be expected to perform for that same person compared to one of these therapies?

To date, neither conventional nor integrative practitioners have a complete set of answers to these questions, although opinions and biases abound. Especially tough are head-to-head comparisons between different methods that are highly dependent on the technique, experience, and skill of the practitioner. Nonetheless, the healing arts are striving to examine these issues with the goal of establishing reasonable recommendations that neither overpromise nor excessively seek to limit the use of a treatment that might benefit certain people.

CAM AND INTEGRATIVE METHODS

One way to sort through the many different methods is to consider them in groups. Within each grouping, interested health-care consumers and those interested in self-care can find methods that appeal to them along with other alternatives that might be worth investigating at another time.

Some integrative methods straddle one or more fields. For example, acupressure can be viewed as an energy therapy as well as a manual or touch therapy. Understanding that some of the methods below could overlap with other fields, the main integrative health categories are:

- Mind-body approaches
- Bodywork and manual therapies
- Natural products
- Traditional healing or whole systems of care
- Energy medicine or bioenergetics

Now let's take a closer look at the different types of methods, with more detailed discussions of many of these specific therapies to follow in subsequent chapters.

Mind-Body Approaches

Mind and body practices use different techniques that are meant to help recruit the power of the mind to influence the function and health of the body or overall health.

Examples of mind-body approaches include meditation, hypnosis, biofeedback, guided imagery, and relaxation therapies such as the relaxation response, a type of deep relaxation behavioral therapy.

Spirituality and prayer may also be considered a mind-body type of approach to healing and well-being. Similar, nonreligious activities such as participation in support groups or in some types of behavioral modification therapy can constitute mind-body interventions.

Mind-body approaches may also have a prominent physical component. Examples of mind-body methods that are integrated with body movement include tai chi, qi gong, and yoga.

Some mind-body methods overlap with those that claim to harness, shift, or transfer energy. Sometimes known as bioenergetics or energy medicine, these other techniques include therapeutic touch, Reiki, magnetic therapy, and sensorial therapies that focus on one or more of the senses such as color therapy, aromatherapy, and music therapy. Acupuncture and its related disciplines may also be considered to make up a special category of energy healing.

Clearly, mind-body approaches can appeal to many different types of people who may have a variety of conditions. For overall health and wellness, individuals may consider mind-body approaches to enhance their overall well-being, sense of connectedness, or inner peace.

Stress-related conditions can be very well served by various mind-body methods. Beyond anxiety, insomnia, and other conditions with strong connections to our emotions and the ways we process information and stress, other conditions may also be responsive to mind-body methods. These can include high blood pressure, headache, traumatic stress disorders, substance abuse, and eating disorders, among others.

Many people incorporate mind-body methods into daily living as a way of bringing tranquility, balance, or inner vitality to their lives. In traditional healing systems such as Ayurveda and traditional Asian healing, meditation and other mind-body methods play a prominent role.

Although mind-body methods can involve deep concentration, relaxation, or other inwardly directed mental energy, many mind-body techniques can also be successfully used in groups for those who prefer to engage with other like-minded individuals. Just as they may be followed in private or as an individual pursuit, modalities such as yoga, tai chi, and even hypnosis and meditation can involve group participation.

Certain mind-body approaches such as meditation or yoga may require repeated practice and training before their benefits can be fully realized. For this reason, it may be preferable to locate an instructor or a group to get started on the right track. Alternatively, many online resources and different media such as DVDs, apps, and books provide other good ways to learn and practice these techniques in private.

Methods such as hypnosis, guided imagery, and biofeedback are best explored with the guidance of a trained professional, at least in the beginning. In later chapters, you will find resources that will help you learn more about these methods and help you locate qualified practitioners.

Mind Over Matter?

Mind-body approaches harness the connectivity between our physical and mental selves. Certain methods such as acupuncture or meditation are long-standing traditions that were passed down over many centuries, long before science had the tools or the need to explain just how such methods might work. Today, we have a better, although still very incomplete, understanding of the mechanisms by which such approaches work in healing or in bringing tranquility to wellness.

The science behind many mind-body techniques includes pathways that kick-start the release of chemicals from the brain and the effects of these chemicals within the cells of the body. Endorphins are a prime example of the body's own "feel-good" chemicals. Once released by the brain, endorphins block or lessen the perception of pain and instead produce an energized feeling or euphoria. Exercise is known to help the body pump out endorphins, which are believed to be responsible for the "runner's high" or other positive feelings associated with physical activity.

Exciting research is beginning to uncover ways that mind-body approaches can have profound effects down to the gene and molecular level. Studies also show that by recruiting the power of the mind, we can override some connections that were once considered hardwired.

Through this modern lens, our brains and internal wiring are seen as being more plastic and changeable than as being fixed at birth or during childhood. These studies also point to our ability to influence or partly regulate some of the systems once thought to be automatic, or running in the background, and thus mostly not controllable. Examples include the stress or "fight or flight" response that helps to preserve the species but can also be harmful when triggered too easily or too often, or when it is stuck in overdrive. Mind-body approaches can be particularly useful in many of these types of stress-related illnesses and conditions.

Some of the conditions or situations that have been helped or treated with mind-body approaches are given below. Because the level of evidence for each method will vary with the condition for which treatment is being sought, discuss your options and preferences with your practitioner to find a safe, effective method that you will be able to follow or participate in to get the best possible benefit. Also, examine which therapy is best suited to your individual concerns and lifestyle, thereby enabling successful and sustainable integration into your overall plan for health.

Conditions That May Benefit from Mind-Body Interventions

- Headache
- Cancer care
- Asthma
- Heart conditions
- Substance abuse
- Epilepsy
- Irritable bowel syndrome
- Stress management
- Hot flashes
- Fibromyalgia
- Inflammation
- Mood, anxiety, depression, and psychiatric disorders
- Chronic pain
- High blood pressure
- Insomnia, sleep disorders
- Eating disorders
- Tinnitus (ringing in the ears)
- Raynaud's disease
- Stroke
- Anxiety or stress before and after surgery
- Concentration or intimacy concerns
- Immune conditions

Bodywork and Manual Therapies

Bodywork and manual therapies involve hands-on approaches that can be designed to relieve physical discomfort but may also involve a mind-body component through relaxation and the easing of stress.

The wide variety of available manual methods will suit a range of personal comfort levels. For individuals who prefer limited touch or minimal disrobing, special touch therapies—such as foot acupressure—or specific bodywork—such as neck massage or spinal manipulation—can be helpful. Many of these different methods are discussed in Chapter 8.

Massage is one of the most popular integrative therapies. Therapeutic massage usually addresses some type of physical or somatic issue, such as back sprain, neck pain and stiffness, or post-athletic muscle soreness and strain. Some types of therapeutic massage can benefit conditions that are also well served by a mind-body approach, such as chronic stress, anxiety, insomnia, or certain digestive disorders. An integrative approach from among the different methods available could be considered in these situations. Massage can also be used to enhance overall health and wellness.

Like other bodywork techniques, massage may involve rubbing, pressing, or otherwise manipulating parts of the body. A therapist may use the hands, elbows, feet, or other areas to stroke or massage the tender part or to work a large part of the body. With techniques such as Rolfing or types of Chinese massage, deep stimulation using the knees or knuckles may also be applied.

Specific types of massage techniques include the following, with general examples of each practice noted below:

- **Swedish massage:** A gentler type of massage that uses lighter, long, and gliding strokes; tapping; gentle kneading; and circular movements of the hands.
- **Sports, deep tissue, or therapeutic massage:** Targeted or more intense massage therapy that involves deeper, firmer, or longer strokes against the muscle grain. This type of massage therapy is often used to address sore spots or activity-related areas such as hamstrings and forearms in tennis players.
- **Chinese massage (tui na):** An ancient technique that also uses pressure, kneading, and other powerful hand techniques applied to specific points of the body to release, restore, or realign energy or *qi*.

Other types of bodywork include the following:

- **Reflexology:** Massage of the feet using the hands or props such as balls or rubber bands. Beyond relaxation, the precise stimulation of certain areas of the feet through reflexology is claimed to affect distant organs, energy flows, or conditions.
- **Feldenkrais:** A method that teaches body awareness and purposeful movements to help improve posture; develop greater flexibility; and foster new patterns of movement, physical transfers (as in from a seated to standing position), and rest.
- **Alexander technique:** Usually taught one-on-one, this method teaches greater body efficiency, awareness, and improved alignment.

In addition to manipulation, osteopaths and chiropractors may also incorporate some type of bodywork in their practice.

- **Chiropractic manipulation**, also known as an adjustment, often involves the practitioner applying a strong yet controlled forceful maneuver to a joint or a section of the body that is designed to improve function or alignment or to decrease stiffness, spasm, or pain.
- **Osteopathic manipulation** is generally less sudden, less high-force, and gentler than a chiropractic adjustment, although it also may involve pressure and stretching without the "cracking" often associated with chiropractic.

Bodywork Benefits and Cautions

Choices among different kinds of bodywork range from techniques that are soothing and comforting to those that can be abrupt or intense, or that vigorously target a problem area of the body. Most massage methods are largely passive for the recipient, whereas Alexander or Feldenkrais methods require more participation on the part of the client in learning new techniques and body awareness.

Work That Body: Safety Tips

Whether you seek bodywork for pleasure and wellness or for a condition that causes you pain or disability, a few cautions apply.

1. Do your homework. Find a trained, experienced, and reputable practitioner who is licensed or certified to practice his or her art.
2. Avoid massage or deeper therapies until any wounds, fractures, dislocations, muscle tears, or skin breaks have healed.
3. Reconsider the chosen type of therapy if you are prone to bleeding, fainting, or dizziness; have fragile bones; or are taking blood thinners.
4. Thoroughly consider the safety or selection of the best therapy with your doctor if you are recovering from surgery, are undergoing cancer care, or are pregnant.

Natural Products

Store shelves at your local pharmacy or big-box stores are overflowing with a wide range of products—from amino acids to botanicals, vitamins, probiotics, and a vast array of supplements, with more coming down the pipeline. Not surprisingly, the use of natural products was the leading CAM method in the U.S., according to the 2012 National Health Interview Survey.

Used for a wide range of ailments as well as for dietary deficiencies, illness prevention, and overall wellness, natural products are used alone or in combination with other integrative therapies. People who are taking prescription medicines also use these products.

Usually taken by mouth, natural products are sold in a variety of forms such as pills, gelcaps, capsules, powders, tinctures, teas, liquids, and concentrates. While most are ready-made and available for off-the-shelf purchase, some natural products are customized, combined, or tailored for an individual's specific condition—a practice that is common in traditional systems of care such as traditional Chinese medicine or Ayurveda.

As discussed in Chapter 3, dietary supplements are classified as a special category of food and do not undergo the approval process for safety and effectiveness that governs prescription medicines before they hit the shelves and are marketed to the general public. Even though gaps and unknowns still exist in the safety profile and usefulness of many of these products, they remain popular choices for self-care.

Because some natural products can have effects on the body similar to the effects caused by prescription drugs, discuss any natural products that you are using with your health-care team. Numerous unanswered questions remain regarding the safety and effectiveness of many, if not most, nonvitamin, nonmineral over-the-counter dietary supplements. Rigorous or long-term information about their safety and usefulness for specific conditions is often lacking, no matter how artfully this information may be disguised on the label or in advertising materials.

Besides, many products interact with each other, with other prescription drugs you may be taking, or with foods. Pharmacists are often available to discuss these issues with you wherever you purchase natural products. You can find more specific information about supplement products in Chapter 9.

Traditional Medicine or Whole Systems of Care

These healing methods and practices are typically steeped in traditions that may go back thousands of years. Examples include Ayurveda, Tibetan medicine, Native American medicine, traditional Chinese medicine (TCM), and other forms of traditional healing. Sometimes called whole systems of care, these therapies are typically focused on healing or wellness that considers the whole person in the holistic context of their society and family, embracing many different types of methods to reach the desired health goal.

For example, the care plan for a person under the care of a TCM practitioner might include a combination of meditation, movement therapy, acupuncture, and different herbs. A person from another village who is evaluated by the same Chinese doctor and who has similar ailments might receive a very different tailored combination of therapies.

Two other types of care are often considered alongside traditional whole systems of care, even though their traditions are not as long-standing and may include a variety of treatments borrowed from different disciplines.

Homeopathy, originally developed in Germany in the late 1700s, is based on two main concepts. Both are at odds with most mainstream medical beliefs. One is the idea that "like cures like," or the law of similars by which a tiny amount of a substance—which, at a higher dose or exposure, can be expected to cause disease in a normal person—can be used to effect a cure. The second major underpinning of homeopathy is that miniscule to nearly undetectable amounts of active ingredients can actually be strong enough to cause desirable effects through cycles of dilutions and shaking known as "potentiation."

Consumers interested in homeopathy should know that unlike dietary supplements that fall under the Dietary Supplement Health and Education Act of 1994, homeopathic medicines have been regulated in the U.S. since 1938 under the federal Food, Drug, and Cosmetic Act. Although homeopathic medicines are not overseen or tested in the same way as prescription drugs, homeopathic product ingredients must be approved by the Homeopathic Pharmacopoeia Convention of the United States (HPCUS), which nevertheless does not ensure that the product will be effective or that it has been shown to be effective.

In addition to prescription homeopathic medicines, nonprescription homeopathic products are also sold over the counter like dietary supplements. Because homeopathic medicines contain miniscule amounts of active ingredients, most are considered safe. However, as with any other CAM therapy, the choice of a homeopathic option for an illness instead of a proven therapy that has been verified to be safe and effective can render what appears to be a safe or natural choice as perhaps unwise compared to what might be gained using a proven treatment.

Naturopathy is another whole system of care that borrows from a variety of practices. Also relatively new, naturopathy is based on a set of principles that embrace the care of the whole person. Naturopathic care aims to do no harm and is focused on patient education and forging a strong doctor-patient relationship. Naturopathy also considers the healing power of nature and, like osteopathic care, places emphasis on prevention. Naturopathic treatments can involve the use of various supplements or other methods such as acupuncture, special diets, and bodywork or physical activity. Some practices also involve different types of injection treatments and, in certain circumstances, prescription medications. These practices are described in greater detail in Chapter 10.

CHOOSING THE BEST PRACTICE METHOD FOR YOU

Because of the abundance of methods out there, choosing the integrative methods that best suit you and will best serve your health can be a challenge.

Those seeking more comprehensive or holistic care may find that whole systems of care, such as naturopathy or TCM, will better suit their needs than more directed or narrow therapies, such as massage or a specific botanical product. On the other hand, people who are generally content with their state of health but who are temporarily suffering from a condition such as neck pain after a whiplash injury may be more interested in a focused approach.

Other considerations to factor into your ultimate choice include where you live and what types of practitioners are available in your community, and whether such providers are reputable or possess the desired licensure. In many communities of the Midwest, Pennsylvania, and California, it can be easier to find a qualified acupuncturist or an osteopath—elsewhere, perhaps not so much.

Insurance considerations also can present problems or opportunities. Millions of Americans pay for CAM out of pocket. According to 2007 statistics, these out-of-pocket expenses totaled nearly $34 billion, accounting for 11% of overall out-of-pocket health-care expenses. With perhaps little or no insurance coverage available, the total cost of treatment and the length of the proposed treatment should also be considered before you determine whether a care path is sustainable for you.

Many insurance plans offer some degree of coverage for certain integrative therapies, including acupuncture. Certain plans require referral by a physician for coverage or may limit coverage to a certain number of visits. Find out what you can expect before embarking on a course of care that may be lengthy or financially burdensome.

Also consider your own personality and tolerance with respect to an integrated plan of care. Are you a get-it-done personality who favors quicker fixes, or are you more comfortable going slow and steady? A quick fixer or someone who prefers to take medications over making long-term lifestyle changes might prefer a supplement over a series of bodywork sessions to help address musculoskeletal problems. Another person who views health and wellness as a journey might prefer the more broad-based and holistic approach of a naturopath or might consider yoga.

At the other end of the spectrum are individuals who thrive on more one-to-one contact with their practitioner and who relish the empowerment that comes with being an engaged pupil, as with learning certain movement therapies. Others still seek more self-directed, action-oriented change, whether through learning new behaviors or relaxation techniques; achieving greater body awareness; or improving the quality of their diet, sleep, and stress-management routines. Older adults or retired persons may find a new sense of social connectedness by participating in integrative group therapies, such as tai chi, that are focused on pain reduction or improving mobility.

Perhaps certain methods or approaches that have been touched on here are already out of the question for you. The lack of a comfort level about needles could stand in the way of acupuncture for some people (even though other related options are available, as discussed in Chapter 6). Others may not feel at ease with massage or may not relish the prospect of having their neck "cracked." The controversies or latest recall regarding dietary supplements, or the uncertainty regarding their usefulness, may also present barriers for certain individuals interested in exploring natural remedies.

Finally, the time commitment for certain treatments also deserves some thought. While little time or effort is spent purchasing and consuming supplements, embarking on a stress-reduction program, following a lengthy chiropractic treatment plan, or pursuing lifestyle modifications to improve heart health can involve a sustained commitment of time and effort.

When embarking on an integrative care plan, be open to reassessing your progress while you decide whether your chosen treatment is indeed the right one for you. Understand that the state of evidence for any given therapy or condition may become stronger or weaker as emerging studies help to refine our beliefs about what works and what might work well enough for your condition and situation.

Above all, you should be comfortable with the skill level, treatments, and care plan provided by your practitioner. Ideally, feedback and communication between you and your entire care team should be a cornerstone of your care, ensuring that you are empowered to reach your health goals in a timely, safe, and nurturing manner.

WHERE TO LEARN MORE

To learn more about the different methods discussed in this chapter, see the specific chapters covering each method and the references provided at the end of each chapter.

6

Acupuncture and Traditional Chinese Medicine

Traditional Chinese medicine and related traditional Asian practices are whole systems of care that integrate a range of methods in accord with long-held beliefs and practices that have evolved over thousands of years.

To simplify the discussion, we will use the term **traditional Chinese medicine**, or TCM, to refer to these non-Western beliefs and practices, understanding that variations exist between how these systems are interpreted and used in Korea, Japan, and other Asian cultures.

In TCM, the body and health are envisioned through concepts, energies, and balance—unlike the Western system that breaks the body down into moving parts or chemicals that work more like a machine, a chemical reaction, or a factory, rather than as an ecosystem.

As a result, the methods used in the diagnosis of conditions and illnesses in TCM often are dramatically different from those associated with mainstream medicine. Adapting to TCM principles requires a different vocabulary and divergent approaches to health and healing that are inviting to certain individuals, but may seem puzzling or unfamiliar to others.

NOT MERELY OF THIS WORLD: UNDERSTANDING TCM

One way to begin to understand TCM is through the idea of inner balance. In Western medicine, it is common to view the body as machinery with inner parts represented by the anatomic structures that we know as organs and organ systems. When these parts wear down or stop working properly, Western medicine offers new parts, such as total joint replacement or new heart valves; spot fixes, such as surgery to improve urine flow in men with enlarged prostates; and medicines that might improve the function of these worn-down parts, such as insulin replacement for diabetics.

In contrast to the mechanical view, TCM perceives the body more like a garden, functioning in health and disease as an interdependent ecosystem rather than as a machine. Health and well-being are seen as states of inner harmony and balance both within the individual and between that person and the outside environment, nature, or the universe. Internal organs are not viewed as parts but rather in terms of their energy. Essential to the health of this inner garden is the fundamental balance and unity of opposite forces or energies. According to TCM, illness is believed to result from an imbalance between these and other forces.

Whereas mainstream medicine may be moving increasingly toward a more holistic approach in assessing an individual's health-care needs, TCM considers the evaluation of the whole being as fundamental. Like its Daoist underpinning, TCM views the person as inherently interconnected to the universe, with internal forces or energy bridging and flowing across both sides. These forces depend on and interact with the other for balance (health) or may shift into imbalance (disease). Interested readers who are intrigued by these concepts may wish to explore other sources to learn more about these complex perspectives.

TCM: ESSENTIAL CONCEPTS

The key concepts underlying much of TCM in principle and practice are those of yin and yang along with the theories of the Five Elements. (Note that we capitalize each of the Five Elements here to denote TCM concepts, not their conventional Western meanings.) These Five Elements are Earth, Fire, Metal, Water, and Wood.

We can better understand yin and yang from our Western perch by looking at nature itself: night versus day, up versus down, and even boy versus girl.

To understand yin and yang from an Oriental view, consider the circle and the square. To Westerners, a circle is just that: It is a circle and not a square and vice-versa—end of discussion. In TCM, a circle can be seen as something that harbors a square within or vice-versa. In other words, the circle has the ability or potential of being a square, with the reverse being that the square is an alternative outline of a circle. This simple example shows us how in TCM, there is less emphasis on reducing interpretations to discrete categorical things and objects. Rather, TCM is focused on the flows and interconnectivity among all things and life itself.

Cold, passive, and dark forces are contained within yin, whereas brighter, warmer, and more expressive forces reign in yang. Because we all have different amounts of these energies inside of us at one time or another, imbalances of yin and yang are viewed in TCM as symptoms of too much Heat (yang) or Cold (yin) that demand different therapies to realign the unsettled forces toward balance.

Another key concept is that of the Five Elements, which are considered as dynamic forces that morph and move within our changing natural world and within our bodies, with all making up the essential parts of a greater, universal system. In TCM, each of the Five Elements of Earth, Fire, Metal, Water, and Wood corresponds to certain tissues of the body, tastes, emotions, yin and yang organs, and other interrelationships and cycles. It is a complex, expansive vision of health.

At the core of traditional Chinese medicine is the energy concept of **qi** (which is sometimes capitalized—Qi), the bioenergy or life force that courses throughout our bodies and the universe. When qi (pronounced *chee*) is in balance, we are healthy and enjoy a sense of well-being. However, when qi stagnates, sinks, is deficient, or flows in the wrong direction, this disharmony is reflected as illness. Disturbances of qi may also be reflected in conditions such as depression or behaviors such as expressing excessive anger.

THE VARIED METHODS OF TCM

Even at an elementary level of understanding, it becomes obvious that appreciating TCM involves a novel point of view regarding how our bodies function, react, and interact with the world around us. Thus, it should come as no surprise that TCM therapies often require a multipronged approach to bring us back to balance and restoration. Concepts such as Blood stagnation or the effects of certain foods or herbs, which can seem unfamiliar or puzzling to mainstream physicians, take on significant meaning to a classically trained doctor of TCM or an acupuncturist.

In TCM healing practices, a range of methods is typically brought into play to reclaim balance and achieve harmony. These modalities can include acupuncture; customized herbal remedies, tinctures, or tonics; massage; meditation; and restorative Asian movement therapies such as qi gong and tai chi (see the next chapter for information about these and other movement methods).

Chinese herbalism is a highly complex field that is nearly always taught in conjunction with acupuncture in China, although not always in the United States. Herbs may be prepared as powders, teas, or tinctures (mixed with a precise amount of water and alcohol to extract the herb's essences) or may be offered raw. Certain classic combinations have been patented for use for a variety of conditions, including menstrual conditions, insomnia, nausea, exhaustion, and respiratory problems.

Despite progress as a result of recent cleanups and improvements in their manufacturing processes, many Chinese herbal products sold in the United States and abroad have been found to contain prescription drugs, substances such as steroids that were not declared on the label, and even toxins—including heavy metals.

Whether patented or not, it is difficult for the health-care consumer to know what is recommended or safe from product to product and producer to producer, and at what dose. Look for certification of good manufacturing practices (GMP) on the label, even though this is not a strict assurance of quality, safety, or effectiveness. (For more information about the regulation and safety of botanicals and dietary supplements, see Chapters 3 and 9.)

Despite the integral part that Chinese herbalism plays in rendering traditional Chinese medical care, the use of these herbs should be guided by caution, especially when their use is considered in at-risk populations such as children, pregnant women, older adults, and people with complex medical conditions or those who take a number of prescription and/or over-the-counter medications and supplements.

AN IN-DEPTH LOOK AT ACUPUNCTURE

Acupuncture, a traditional Oriental practice that continues to gain in acceptance and is more widely used among Americans considering integrative care, is a long-standing healing method that has been used for thousands of years. While the history of acupuncture can be traced to ancient China, recent findings from studies of our primitive ancestors have suggested that the use of acupuncture may extend even further, perhaps as many as 5,000—or more—years ago.

Acupuncture involves the superficial insertion of hair-thin needles at certain points of the body called **acupoints**. When practiced by a trained and skilled practitioner using sterile needles, acupuncture has been shown to be not only safe but also effective for a variety of ailments such as various types of pain, arthritis, and headache, among others. The use of acupuncture appears encouraging for a growing range of conditions, with varying evidence levels of effectiveness for an expanding number of health problems (see Table 1 on page 87).

With growing evidence for its usefulness, its wide availability, and the fact that acupuncture is easily accessible and has an excellent safety profile compared to many conventional treatments, more people are becoming interested in exploring acupuncture. According to the last national health statistical report to examine acupuncture in 2012, close to 4 million American adults have experienced acupuncture. Most surveyed Americans sought acupuncture for lower back pain, followed by joint pain, neck pain, and headaches, including migraines. With more conventional and integrative practitioners and consumers gaining familiarity and comfort with acupuncture, these numbers are certain to grow.

Getting the Point

Acupuncture was unfamiliar to most Americans until reporter James Reston wrote about his unexpected acupuncture experience in a 1971 front-page *New York Times* article, "Now, Let Me Tell You About My Appendectomy in Peking...." Reston, who was attempting to interview Mao Tse-tung, then Chairman of the Communist Party of China, on the day that Secretary of State Henry Kissinger secretly arrived as a prelude to President Richard Nixon's groundbreaking China visit, became ill with appendicitis. After his appendix was removed at the Anti-Imperialist Hospital while he was under local anesthesia, he experienced a great deal of pain and fullness. A young acupuncturist who was not a medical doctor performed acupuncture on Reston, using burning herbs for heat, all of which appeared rather odd to the inquisitive reporter. Reston was reassured that the stimulation provided by acupuncture could help relieve or unblock the congestion that was causing his pain and bloat. When it did, Reston told the world about China's ancient method, just as that country began its rise to global prominence, which brought acupuncture onto the radar of Americans and other Westerners.

What Is Acupuncture?

According to traditional Chinese medicine and other Asian healing traditions, acupoints at the surface of the body represent areas that are connected to our deeper organ systems and energy flows. Acupuncturists target these specific points to redirect or restore energy, or to correct imbalances that are believed to be causing the disorder that prompts a patient to seek treatment.

The aim of acupuncture is to aid in the restoration of inner balance. This is accomplished by the placement of acupuncture needles at very specific areas that correspond to certain energy points. In TCM, the different acupoints mark connection points to the energy flows within the body that travel along 14 **meridians**, or energy pathways.

As described earlier, this bioenergy network that powers our vitality largely rests on a balance between the opposing forces of yin and yang. Other points that an acupuncturist stimulates may not correspond to a specific meridian but may relate instead to a sensitive or tender spot, known as **Ashi** points.

Illness, from the viewpoint of people who follow TCM, results from a blockage or obstruction of qi. By stimulating, opening, reversing, or releasing the flow of energy through the precise placement of acupuncture needles, the acupuncturist seeks to help bring patients back to balance and to restore their vital flows of inner bioenergy.

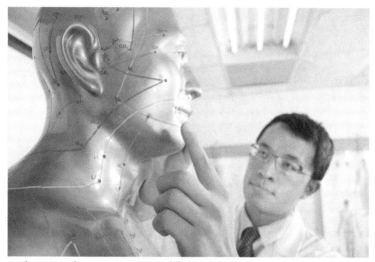

A physician demonstrates a model showing various body acupoints and meridians.

If you are curious about acupuncture or have decided to pursue an acupuncture treatment for a specific health goal or relieve a painful condition, it is not required for you to understand or to accept the broader teachings of TCM or other belief systems. For many people and their health providers, acupuncture is only one of many treatment methods used to promote health and counter illness. You should feel at ease when approaching an acupuncturist for the first time and feel empowered to understand, accept, or reject treatments other than acupuncture that you may be offered.

Still, an appreciation of certain TCM concepts can help you gain a better understanding of what acupuncture involves. This knowledge can help you decide whether acupuncture, or acupuncture in combination with another traditional method such as movement therapy or meditation, might be right for you.

How Does Acupuncture Work?

Doctors of Oriental Medicine (OMDs and others) understand acupuncture to work according to traditional beliefs and concepts. The practice of acupuncture has also been studied from a Western scientific perspective. Although this method of inquiry is sometimes viewed as reductionist, it also serves a purpose. These studies tell us that when acupuncture stimulates small nerves within muscles, these nerves send signals that travel to different parts of the nervous system within the spinal cord and deep into the brain. In turn, the relayed signals cause the release of certain chemical substances or neurochemicals such as norepinephrine, a stimulant, and endorphins, which are substances with calming effects that counteract the sensation of pain to produce a feeling of well-being or bliss.

Acupuncture also triggers the release of certain messaging substances called neurotransmitters as well as hormones that stimulate the adrenal gland to make cortisol, a hormone with known anti-inflammatory effects. This may be one way that acupuncture helps in the treatment of inflammatory conditions such as arthritis or fibromyalgia.

Hey Iceman, Where'd Ya Get That Tattoo?

In 1991, hikers discovered a 5,300-year-old mummified man in the ice and snow of the Italian Alps. Named Ötzi for the mountains where he was found along with much of his clothing and possessions, the Tyrolean Iceman is one of the world's most important historical discoveries. While other mummies that harbor tattoos have been found, Ötzi's tattoos were different. Many of his markings that were not decorations were located on areas of his skin that were not believed to be exposed, prompting researchers to ask whether they might have had ritualistic or medicinal meaning. After a curious acupuncturist determined that many of Ötzi's markings corresponded to known acupoints, an analysis by experts from three European acupuncture societies concluded that at least nine of Ötzi's markings were within six millimeters of acupoints. A few other markings on the mummy were only slightly farther away from other acupoints. These markings corresponded to acupoints that could have been used to treat back and other joint pain, which correlated with X-ray findings that indicated joint disease in Ötzi's hips, knees, and spine. These discoveries suggested that acupuncture, believed to have been used in China for at least 2,000 years, might have been used for much longer and perhaps had a Eurasian footprint as well.

Locally, acupuncture also increases blood flow to the site being needled, thereby bringing added nutrients and oxygen to that area. Recent studies have also shown that acupuncture may also exert its beneficial effects by influencing gene expression—the ways that certain genes function, behave, or regulate or control certain activities at a nuclear or cellular level.

What to Expect During Your Visit

Because the type of professional training varies between different types of licensed acupuncturists, a visit to a physician acupuncturist may be quite different from a visit to an OMD or an acupuncturist who was trained in traditional Asian medicine.

Also, if you were referred to an acupuncturist from your conventional provider for an already diagnosed or specific ailment such as lower back pain, the acupuncturist may focus primarily on delivering the treatment alone rather than on the performance of an extensive diagnostic examination. The acupuncturist also might not suggest other complementary approaches for your condition, such as meditation or movement therapy.

Traditional acupuncturists generally perform a visual inspection, which often includes examination of the tongue, hands, and other areas. Classically trained acupuncturists also take into account pulse diagnosis, a method used to assess wellness or disease by thoughtful examination of your pulse beyond merely its rate. Whichever type of practitioner you visit, describe your health problem in your own words to guide the acupuncturist in tailoring a treatment approach that is suited to your specific condition.

Treatment is usually rendered in a clean, private, and quiet room where you will be allowed to loosen your clothing and lie down. The acupuncturist will feel any areas to be needled, whether on your legs, arms, head, or elsewhere. After cleansing the skin, you will first feel light pressure as the acupuncturist seats a small hollow tube or introducer over the area to be needled. Once the sterile, single-use needle has been unwrapped and dropped into the tube, the acupuncturist will either gently tap the needle or advance it, inserting it into the skin to the desired depth. Some acupuncturists do not use an introducer and simply insert the needle and tap it into place, as is often done with ear (auricular) acupuncture. Typically, the needle is advanced no more than an inch and is often closer to one-quarter inch.

You might feel a light pinch or pressure, but because the needles are very thin, most people generally do not report unpleasantness or pain. The practitioner will gently advance the needle until it is properly secured by the tissues or until the patient experiences a sensation of heaviness or fullness known as **de qi**, which means the arrival of qi. The number of needles used will vary with the condition and the acupoint sites. Most treatments require the placement of between five and 15 needles.

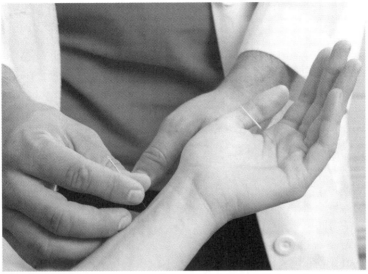

An acupuncturist inserts a sterile acupuncture needle into the arm.

Once all of the needles have been placed, the acupuncturist may leave the room to allow you to lay still for about half an hour or longer, often with soft music playing and the lights dimmed. This is a time to relax or meditate, and to avoid focusing on anything that makes your anxious—your to-do list for the day, worries, or negative thoughts—and to concentrate instead on healing and mindfulness.

Afterwards, the acupuncturist will quickly remove each needle, another step that is most commonly pain-free and uneventful. Unlike having your blood drawn through a much larger needle, there is usually no need to apply pressure to the needled points. The acupuncturist will typically ask how you are feeling and allow you to slowly bring yourself to a comfortable seated position before you are asked to stand. Finally, provided all has gone well and you are comfortable, you will be permitted to return to your daily activities.

Side effects from acupuncture are exceedingly rare. Although some serious events such as bleeding or unintended puncture have been reported, when used appropriately by a trained practitioner, the procedure is considered one of the safest treatments available. Minor side effects can include pain from the needling, dizziness, and minor bruising. However, in the vast majority of cases, patients view the experience as calming and restorative.

Although rare side effects may still occur in the best of hands, it is important to also keep in mind that the use of acupuncture for painful conditions such as tennis elbow, arthritis, and fibromyalgia is associated with fewer side effects than typical Western medical therapies such as steroid injections and anti-inflammatory medications.

A series of acupuncture visits is usually recommended for long-standing conditions such as joint, neck, or back pain as well as for certain types of headaches. Typically, about ten sessions may be recommended.

People who prefer a treatment that does not involve the use of needles have turned to **acupressure**. In this technique, the acupuncturist examines and assesses the patient as they would for acupuncture and locates the appropriate acupoints for stimulation. However, instead of using thin needles, the acupoints are stimulated by manual pressure.

Many patients are able to learn how to stimulate specific acupoints on themselves, which offers a low-cost and safe way for individuals to deliver self-care for certain conditions, as in the prevention of nausea or motion sickness. Acubands are pressure-sensitive wristbands that can deliver stimulation of an acupoint (acustimulation) when they are worn to obtain the desired therapeutic effects.

For example, stimulation of the wrist acupoint (P6, also known as MH-6 or Master of the Heart 6) has been found to aid in the prevention of motion sickness. This treatment has also been found to work as well as drugs in the prevention of nausea and vomiting that may occur after surgery.

This acupoint can easily be found by placing the second, third, and fourth fingers of your opposite hand together and just below the base of the thumb or at the wrist crease, as shown in the illustration on the next page. With your ring finger at the point where the base of the hand meets the wrist, find the P6 or MH-6 acupoint just to the far side of the index finger, near the base of the fingernail and the creases that mark the farthest joint of the finger.

Two other common variations of acupuncture are Japanese and Korean acupuncture. Although there are many similarities between these two practices and Chinese acupuncture—from which they are derived—Japanese acupuncture relies more on physical examination, a method of touch sensation called palpation. Stimulation in Japanese acupuncture may also be milder and might involve stroking or scratching the skin with the needle instead of inserting it into the skin. In Korean acupuncture, a greater number of needles may be used.

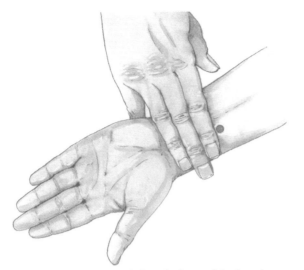

Locate the P6 or MH-6 acupoint below the base of the hand.
Illustration credit: Gabriella Ritts, with permission.

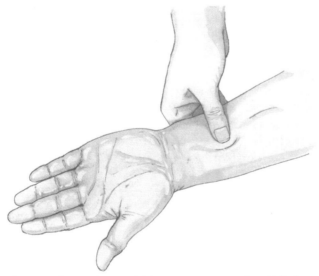

The P6 or MH-6 acupoint to which acupressure can be applied.
Illustration credit: Gabriella Ritts, with permission.

Besides the use of needles, a trained acupuncturist may also stimulate acupoints with heat, as with the burning of a tightly wrapped bunch of the mugwort herb moxa, a technique known as **moxibustion**.

Electroacupuncture is another way to stimulate acupoints using a safe and low voltage of electrical energy, a method that appears to be gaining in popularity. Studies have suggested that electroacupuncture may release our own internal endorphins more consistently than manual acupuncture methods. Some practitioners have incorporated the use of laser in their practices, stimulating acupoints with finely directed beams of laser energy.

Don't Needle Me

Alternative therapies are available for people whose anxiety about needles overshadows their potential interest in acupuncture. With acupressure, the practitioner uses similar diagnostic clues and acupoints to apply manual pressure, but does so without needling. Medical acupuncturists whose training includes the safe use of laser energy can also use lasers instead of needles to stimulate acupoints, with the ear being a frequent target. Laser acupuncture has also been used for childhood conditions, including nighttime bed wetting and asthma.

Cupping is another method that is often used along with acupuncture. As its name implies, cupping involves the placement of a warmed cup or cups on the skin while the patient is at rest and after the acupuncture needles have been placed in position. The upper back is a common site for cupping. As the warmed air inside the cups cools, suction is created, bringing greater blood flow to the areas under the cups. The temporary redness that typically appears after cupping usually resolves within one or two days.

Not to be confused with acupuncture is a new and controversial technique known as **dry needling** that is now being used by some physical therapists. Used for pain relief, this method uses ultrathin needles that are inserted into muscle tissues or trigger points to relieve different types of painful myofascial conditions. The potential harms and benefits of this procedure remain mostly unknown, as there is little experience, long-term follow-up, or detailed scientific investigation into this relatively new technique.

Conditions That May Be Helped by Acupuncture

The World Health Organization (WHO) issued an exhaustive evaluation of randomized **controlled trials** involving acupuncture in 1996 that pointed to the effective use of this therapy in about 30 conditions, ranging from hay fever to stroke and beyond. A year later, a conference held by the National Institutes of Health that examined decades of studies concluded that acupuncture might represent an acceptable alternative treatment for certain conditions or as a therapy to be used alongside other conventional methods. Since then, research into acupuncture has accelerated, and new studies are published worldwide on a daily basis. In 2002, the WHO issued an extensive review and analysis of controlled trials on acupuncture for a host of conditions; this is available on the WHO website link at the end of this chapter.

Large trials in which the use of acupuncture was studied in thousands of people have shown that the benefits of acupuncture are relevant compared with usual care. Some studies have also shown that the results can last for at least six months after treatment. In addition, acupuncture can lessen the use of prescription drugs, can improve quality of life, and may decrease the number of missed workdays due to illness or bothersome conditions. For hundreds of millions of people worldwide, acupuncture is an inexpensive and accessible method of care.

Acupuncture has also been used prominently in emergency situations, as was shown in the aftermath of Hurricane Katrina. The U.S. military has had success with and a growing interest in acupuncture for migraine under duress, sometimes called "battlefield acupuncture."

The body of evidence concerning acupuncture continues to grow and to be refined. Although the conditions listed in Table 1 below are not as exhaustive as those given in the 1996 WHO report, the table includes conditions for which the evidence for acupuncture treatment is strongest in the first column; conditions for which acupuncture is encouraging in the middle column; and conditions for which evidence for acupuncture is low, controversial, or absent in the last column.

However, each individual and situation is different, so consult with your health-care practitioner to find the best solution or combination of treatments for you. The safety, relative affordability, and availability of acupuncture can also be factored in when approaching a decision about using acupuncture for health and wellness.

TABLE 1. CONDITIONS THAT MAY BE HELPED BY ACUPUNCTURE

| | EVIDENCE LEVEL | |
SUPPORTIVE	*MODERATE*	*LOW OR UNCERTAIN*
Arthritis (osteoarthritis)	Dental pain	Irritable bowel syndrome
Nausea and vomiting	Carpal tunnel syndrome	Autism
Headaches (tension, migraine)	Diabetic peripheral neuropathy	Substance abuse/ addiction
Fibromyalgia	Menstrual cramps	Insomnia
Chronic pain	Cancer care symptoms	Epilepsy
Ileus after surgery	Stroke rehabilitation	Traumatic brain injury
Neck/back pain	Asthma (nonacute)	Smoking cessation
Knee osteoarthritis pain	Allergy/sinusitis	

How to Find an Acupuncturist

Many mainstream physicians today are open to referring their patients for acupuncture. Dentists are also among the conventional practitioners who are embracing acupuncture, whether within their practice settings or by referral. Although acupuncture falls within a medical doctor's scope of practice in most states, special training, experience, and licensure in acupuncture are generally required and highly desirable. Physicians can become board certified in acupuncture after training through the American Board of Medical Acupuncture.

If you prefer to see an acupuncturist who is not an M.D. or one who is trained and experienced in traditional Asian techniques, seek a licensed acupuncture practitioner, abbreviated as LAc, or a Doctor of Oriental Medicine. To practice acupuncture and traditional Asian medicine, most states require certification from the National Certification Commission for Acupuncture and Oriental Medicine (NCCAOM).

Besides acupuncture, the NCCAOM also awards diplomates in Chinese herbology and Asian bodywork therapy. Typically, someone who holds an NCCAOM diplomate of acupuncture has received three to four years of training at the master's degree level at an accredited acupuncture program. These practitioners typically are trained in and may treat a greater variety of acupoints than other types of health-care professionals who have received more limited acupuncture training, such as chiropractors, naturopaths, and mainstream medical doctors and nurses.

To achieve certification as a Doctor of Acupuncture and Oriental Medicine (DAOM), the applicant must first attain master's level training (for example, a Master's of Science in Oriental Medicine (MSOM)), from an accredited school with on-site course work and training in Chinese herbology. Distance learning is not an acceptable substitution. The NCCAOM website (*nccaom.org*) has helpful information for consumers, a state licensure map, links to accredited schools, and a listing of practitioners.

Know that acupuncture licensure requirements vary from state to state and that the terms used to describe different—or even similar—types of acupuncturists and TCM practitioners can be confusing. For example, some states refer to LAcs as "doctors of oriental medicine," a title that does not necessarily reflect the achievement of an actual doctoral degree.

In addition, even though a master's degree is the minimal, entry-level degree required for graduates of Oriental medicine schools to practice in the United States, the degrees awarded by different acupuncture and Oriental medicine schools can vary in name, as in Master of Science in Traditional Chinese Medicine versus Master of Traditional Oriental Medicine—two degrees that can reflect very similar training.

To confuse matters even further, although degree programs conferring the Oriental Medical Doctor (OMD) were discontinued in the 1990s when the NCCAOM established the master's-based accreditation and degree-granting structure, you may encounter practitioners who use OMD after their name, signifying that they completed their doctoral training program in TCM before 1990.

Acupuncture treatment may be covered by your health insurance. Some policies require a physician referral or specify insurance coverage for only certain conditions or for a maximum number of sessions within a certain time period. What is also worth noting is that many insurers will only allow coverage for treatments rendered by a licensed acupuncturist. Look into your coverage details to determine whether and how many treatments may be covered and what restrictions might apply.

TIPS FOR A SUCCESSFUL ACUPUNCTURE VISIT

Whether you're new to acupuncture or have experienced treatments in the past, follow these tips to ensure a relaxing visit to your acupuncturist. First-time visits may take an hour or slightly longer, so plan accordingly to reap the greatest benefit from the calming and restorative afterglow.

- Eat a light, healthy snack about an hour before you arrive.
- Drink a small glass of water before your appointment time.
- Empty your bladder before you go for treatment or before entering the treatment room.
- Wear loose, comfortable clothing; avoid belts, jewelry, and busy or tight-fitting clothes or snug undergarments.
- Be sure to tell your acupuncturist about any blood thinners or other medications you are taking that could affect blood clotting.
- Let your acupuncturist know if you are experiencing light-headedness, anxiety, or any other condition that might affect the treatment or plan.
- Avoid scheduling intense or stressful activities after your visit—try to rest or stay in the zone after your visit ends.
- Keep yourself well hydrated and enjoy a lighter, nutrient-packed dinner that evening.

WHERE TO LEARN MORE

National Certification Commission for Acupuncture and Oriental Medicine: *www.nccaom.org*

American Academy of Medical Acupuncture: *www.medicalacupuncture.org*

Academic Consortium for Complementary and Alternative Health Care: *www.accahc.org*

World Health Organization: *www.who.int*

The Web That Has No Weaver: Understanding Chinese Medicine by Ted Kaptchuk, 2000.

7

Mind-Body and Energy Therapies

IND-BODY APPROACHES TO HEALTH AND WELLNESS INCLUDE A WIDE RANGE of practices. Despite variations in methods, they have a basic principle in common: the ability of the mind to positively influence physical and overall health. This mind-body connection, which skeptics might brand as wishful thinking or some kind of puffery, has been supported by reams of scientific evidence and actual practice over different facets of everyday life, and in varying states of health and illness.

This chapter includes mind-body and deep relaxation techniques such as meditation and guided imagery, along with methods that have a more prominent physical component such as yoga.

Finally, we'll also explore methods that could otherwise be classified as **bioenergetics**, a term borrowed from biochemistry involving the study of energy transfers and transformation. In integrative health, bioenergetics or energy therapies refer to approaches that enhance, restore, or rebalance the energy within us toward health and wellness. Notable examples include methods such as acupuncture (more fully discussed in Chapter 6) that are supported by a great deal of evidence and those for which evidence is evolving, scanty, or absent, such as magnet therapy.

THE MIND-BODY CONNECTION: AN ANTIDOTE TO STRESS

Stress was once considered an annoying but benign aspect of life's ups and downs—something to get over, forget about, or power through. We now know that stress, especially chronic types of stress that persist over time without relief, can be harmful in many ways—and even deadly.

Our bodies are designed to respond positively to certain stresses. Among these reactions is the "fight or flight" response, which is innately present in humans and many other living creatures. The "fight or flight" reaction is triggered when we perceive a threat of some kind that must be avoided. When our brain receives signals from our body, eyes, nose, or other sensory organs that relay danger, our bodies respond on multiple levels. These responses allow us to call up the strength and resources to fight the threat or to flee quickly away from it.

Included in these stress reactions is an outpouring of stress hormones such as adrenaline (from the adrenal glands), along with brain chemicals known as **neurotransmitters** that help put the brain and nervous system on maximum alert. While all of this is happening, a series of events occur.

Breathing patterns shift, and our bronchial breathing tubes expand to allow the body to take in more oxygen. Our pupils dilate, allowing us to take in more visual cues. Meanwhile, the heart speeds up, thumping into overdrive to quickly pump more higher-pressure, oxygen-rich blood to tissues like muscles that need that extra burst of energy to fight or take flight. With the help of certain nerves, blood is shifted away from digestive centers and the skin and moves toward the muscles and organs that are vital to sustaining the stress response. Even the hair on our skin is affected by the stress response, signifying alertness by standing on end.

Normally, once the stress passes, our systems reset, going back to their prestress state of normalcy or balance. Stress chemicals that were released are swept up, and different, calming chemicals are released, restoring balance.

However, for a variety of reasons, the stress response doesn't completely turn off or remains chronically switched on, as can occur with chronic pain or with certain phobias or fears. Stress can also be associated with treatments or diseases that come on in an unpredictable way and that cause great distress when they are active. Examples include painful migraine headaches or the many disturbing symptoms associated with irritable bowel syndrome or fibromyalgia.

Mind-body therapies are antidotes to stress. Solid scientific studies have shown that by using the mind to calm the body—and, holistically, the entire organism—the stress response described above can be reversed or significantly dialed down all the way to the level of cells and molecules. We are just beginning to uncover the ways in which successful stress management through mind-body therapies can alter the structure and function of the essential material within cell nuclei, the central command stations within our cells, perhaps to the level of DNA itself.

Different mind-body methods can use one or a combination of methods to bring about profound and healing inner calm. Breathing, movement, and mental focus are some of the ways that the healing centers in our brain can be stimulated to release powerful chemicals such as pain-relieving and pleasure-enhancing endorphins. These and other methods can also stimulate certain brain pathways, or the release of neurotransmitters and hormones, that act to calm overly stimulated organs or blood vessels to restore a healthier balance.

Practicing the Relaxation Response

Seat yourself comfortably in a quiet room and try this simple method to tense and then relax your muscles to bring on a relaxation effect. You can also try this in bed if you are having trouble sleeping.

- Flex your foot by pointing your toes toward your body.
- Hold that position for a few seconds, but not to the point of pain.
- Take a deep breath, concentrating on the tension of your flexed foot.
- As you let go of the tension, let out your breath and concentrate mentally on the relaxation itself, saying the word "relax" slowly to yourself or aloud.
- Repeat these steps a few times until the relaxation sensation deepens.

Now that you've begun to relax, we will begin with meditation, a mind-body method that has played a major role in multicultural and spiritual belief systems for thousands of years.

MEDITATION

Meditation is practiced in a variety of ways and for many reasons. Meditation benefits the mind, body, and spirit, a payload that offers a great deal to those who struggle with the pressures of fast-paced modern living. For those who have a less stressful lifestyle or who live in peaceful environments or close to nature, meditation can still offer a path to calm and inner peace.

Despite its practice worldwide, meditation was little known in the U.S. until the 1950s. However, meditation is now widely used. According to a 2008 survey, about one in 10 American adults have had experience with meditation. By 2012 estimates, that's nearly 20 million Americans—not including another million or so youth aged four to 17.

Meditation and The Beatles

Meditation was undiscovered by most Americans during the first half of the 20th century. Then, in the 1950s, India's Maharishi Mahesh Yogi introduced a deep form of meditation to a global audience through stirring tours and best-selling books (*Science of Being and Art of Living*, 1963). When The Beatles spoke and sang about their interest in transcendence, meditation, and the Maharishi himself at the peak of their culture-jolting popularity, a new awareness of meditation and Eastern spiritual traditions swept through America and many parts of the world. Along with this soaring interest came influential trends in music (the sitar) and fashion (Nehru jackets, for better or worse). Words such as "guru" and "mantra" became the totally transcendental language of the times and are now embedded in the lexicon.

Like other mind-body approaches, meditation recruits the power of the mind to influence the function of the body. As a result, meditation practices can affect our mental state, perception, or coping with respect to symptoms that we experience, such as anxiety or pain. Others seek to explore meditation to foster wellness or to support their overall health or performance.

Simply put, meditation is a practice that involves quieting the mind in a way that brings peacefulness, focus, and joy. The result is that the meditator, with practice, reaches a state of profound awareness, insight, and tranquility.

To learn meditation is to learn release from the daily distractions and stresses of modern living. Meditators learn to direct their energy inward instead, gaining and reclaiming focus. With practice, meditators reach a blissful, quiet stillness of compassion and acceptance.

In a sense, it is easier to explain what meditation is not than to explain exactly what it is, especially because many of the words used to describe the process or results of meditation are at odds with what meditation truly involves. Meditation is not about doing an activity, striving to do or achieve something, or fixing things. Meditation is not a method to make your mind go blank or to escape from reality or responsibilities; rather, meditation is about letting go of needs, thoughts, and distractions. By focusing attention on the present, and by redirecting focus to the here and now, the meditator becomes open to mindfulness, embracing the tranquility of the sublime stillness that was profoundly and deeply present all the while.

Meditative tranquility may seem elusive for individuals who follow a no-pain, no-gain or an "I-me-mine" way of life. For the highly scheduled or the more-better-faster crowd, meditative calm may seem downright unreachable. The idea of meditation can also be challenging for less fortunate individuals for whom every day entails another round of struggles to overcome.

Acceptance of meditation can also be iffy for workaholics or people who are on edge or rest-deprived. Finding peace in meditation can also appear undoable to those who are stuck in a reactive mode that requires them to chronically put out fires caused by systems or by loved ones or individuals who are not performing as expected or who are chronically causing trouble. Others might write off meditation as gloomy or something for the self-indulgent, loners, or people of a certain faith.

Yet, all of these types of individuals can benefit from and learn meditation. There are plenty of options you can explore to get you started.

How Does Meditation Work?

In traditional healing systems, meditation is one aspect of a way of life and culture. These healing ways may also include dietary practices and spirituality, among others, which can make it difficult to sort out the isolated or specific effects of meditation on the body or on risk factors for disease.

Taking stock of meditation's benefits can also be hard to measure or to prove using a scientific method. Many studies have aimed to assess how effectively meditation or other integrative practices work compared to other methods, providing useful information for health consumers as well as practitioners.

Nevertheless, controlled and uncontrolled scientific studies have pointed to a variety of ways or mechanisms by which meditation appears to affect and promote health. Among the conditions that have been studied relative to meditation are asthma, allergy and immune conditions, heart and vascular disease, respiratory and gastrointestinal ailments, psychiatric and sexual conditions, substance use disorders, aging, cancer, pain disorders, musculoskeletal problems, and skin conditions.

One way to understand the scientific basis for meditation is to consider yin and yang, the two opposing forces in traditional Chinese medicine. These beliefs hold that our bodies are ruled by opposing internal forces that help regulate how our organs behave. In turn, these forces affect how our bodies function, depending on the need or situation, and the state of health or disease.

Interestingly, with respect to yin and yang, medical science has detailed two counterbalancing domains within our nervous system called the **sympathetic** and the **parasympathetic** nervous systems. The sympathetic system revs up the body and prepares it for action, as occurs with a "fight or flight" encounter, whereas the parasympathetic system helps restore balance by exerting opposite effects.

Studies of meditation have shown effects on both of these systems, providing explanations and an understanding of meditation's effects on the mind-body connection in discrete, scientific terms.

In studies of mindfulness techniques, people who meditated reacted to stresses and provocative events as though those events had been filtered through a different lens. Rather than responding by negative thinking patterns and reactive states, the mindfulness group had more positive, adaptive ways of handling stressful conditions, akin to an outlook that views the glass as half full rather than half empty.

Mindfulness and other meditative practices allowed stresses that might have been seen as obstructions, frightening, or anxiety-provoking to be viewed or reimagined instead as challenges. Defanged, such challenges are met by the meditative mind with hopefulness and optimism-fueled energy for a satisfactory resolution rather than being met with reactivity, anxiety, or anger. In a sense, this process may be seen as a more profound and empowered attitude adjustment.

These effects can be translated in terms of specific body functions. Meditation has been linked to the lowering of blood pressure and to reduced risk factors for diseases of the heart and blood vessels, known as **cardiovascular disease**. Meditation has also been shown to help our hearts maintain a rhythm that follows a healthier, more regular ebb and flow.

Many people consider meditation for heart or vascular health. In 2013, a study group for the American Heart Association concluded that alternative approaches for lowering blood pressure are worth considering as add-on therapies for certain people. While the group found stronger evidence for the effectiveness of exercise for reducing blood pressure than was found for transcendental meditation, yoga, and biofeedback, the scientific statement reported that these latter methods were worthy approaches to consider. Meditation was also supported because it carries a low risk for harm, has the potential for other positive health benefits, and is widely available.

Meditation, Telomeres, and Aging

A recent and exciting discovery notes the positive association of mindfulness meditation and a measurement of cellular aging—telomere length. Telomeres, the protective protein structures that serve as the endcaps of our DNA-containing chromosomes, shorten with advancing age. Telomeres also shorten when cells divide so that eventually, the telomeres are so whittled down that the cell dies. As telomeres shorten, the genetic material inside a cell becomes unstable, which can also lead to cancerous change. An enzyme called telomerase helps certain cells maintain their DNA chromosome length and stability.

Telomeres, the subject of the 2009 Nobel Prize in Physiology or Medicine, are prone to damage by different types of stress. They are shorter in patients with major types of depression; in patients with Alzheimer's disease; and in people who endure chronic and stressful life experiences, such as caregivers and people of low socioeconomic status.

However, meditation and other lifestyle changes have been shown to have positive effects on telomere maintenance and length, as well as on the activity of the telomerase enzyme. It seems that what's good for the telomere is good for the organism.

Types of Meditation

To understand some of the differences among types of meditation, consider these basic practice types, noting that some of the practices overlap.

- Focused meditation
- Mantra meditation
- Faith or spiritual meditation
- Movement meditation

Focused Meditation

Also known as **concentrative meditation**, this practice involves letting go of all thoughts and distractions to exist fully in the moment.

Mindfulness meditation (MM) is a popular example of focused meditation that has been well studied. MM has been shown to aid concentration and to help individuals with coping, stress, and anxiety. Variations that are based on MM include mindfulness-based stress reduction (MBSR) and mindfulness-based cognitive therapy (MBCT).

Of the various meditation methods, mindfulness meditation has been especially brought into the mainstream at health-care facilities, universities, schools, and workplaces across the country. The U.S. military and some professional sports teams also use mindfulness training.

Mindfulness involves learning not just how to pay attention but also how to restore focus and let go of random or intrusive thoughts. That does not mean that we ignore these thoughts, wish them away, or deny that they exist. Rather, mindfulness teaches us to acknowledge such thoughts and, without judging them, to release them and circle back to concentration, whether through breathing, by using a fixed point, or perhaps through the repetition of a sound or word.

The key to mindfulness meditation is becoming focused on being fully present in the moment. With practice, mindfulness can serve as a powerful mental antidote to stressful living. Besides bringing a sense of calm and acceptance, mindfulness and meditation can help you develop more positive ways of coping and can help lessen unproductive, reactive, or repetitive thinking. The act of learning to meditate can also give meditators a better sense of control over wandering thoughts, their health, and stressful life events. Meditation can also help individuals who remain focused on or pained by past hurts or difficulties find forgiveness, release, and peace.

With practice, the meditator no longer hurtles along in a reactive mode to all that swirls around like a pinball off the bumpers. Rather, the meditator becomes enveloped in the fullness of the moment and is free of thoughts and sensation. Upon reaching that point of bliss, the meditator can experience a profound spiritual release that brings a deep sense of connection and strength, both inward to the individual's deepest essence and outward to feel connected with others, life, and—perhaps—universally. Beyond all that we can see, touch, hear, feel, smell, and taste, meditation bridges a connection with the core of existence that binds all forms of life, matter, and metaphysical being.

Vipassanā meditation is another focused-based method. Rooted in ancient Buddhist teachings, Vipassanā features four pillars of mindfulness, beginning with the mindfulness of breathing.

Zen meditation is another focused type of practice with a strong emphasis on the contemplative. A Buddhist meditative practice, Zen (sometimes known as zazen) involves delving deep into and beyond our inner selves to awaken the enlightened self that was always present. Although the roots of Zen began in sixth-century China, Zen has spread and been adopted in Korea, India, Japan, and parts of south Asia, as well as in the West. The practice of Zen often requires a commitment to longer periods of training than mindfulness approaches—from months to many years.

Recommended Reading: *Siddhartha*

In *Siddhartha*, a novel by the German author Hermann Hesse first published in 1922, a young man embarks on a quest of self-discovery. Having left behind his home and family, Siddhartha encounters false paths, rejection, and conflict on this way to experiencing transformational truth and wisdom. This contemplative, lyrical novel is best savored over short reading sessions, allowing the reader to absorb many concepts related to Buddhism, Zen, and the universal obstacles to selfless fulfillment.

Mantra meditations involve the repetition of a word or phrase, whether voiced or not, which may overlap with other types of meditative practice.

The meditator might repeat a word, phrase, or sound, such as the familiar *om* (pronounced *ohm*). The word could also be an affirmation or, in faith-guided meditations, a word or phrase with religious meaning. By directing and refocusing attention to the repeated word or idea, the meditator learns to experience a greater state of awareness or an expanded level of consciousness.

Transcendental meditation is perhaps the best-known type of mantra meditation. Rooted in Hindu origins, this form of meditation can require intensive practice but can also be self-directed. Often, a teacher offers words for the student meditator to repeat (the mantra), which the meditator eventually learns to do effortlessly as transcendence is reached.

Faith and Spiritual Meditation

Different types of meditation have been taught and practiced among ancient tribal cultures and in Eastern traditions such as Buddhism, Taoism, and Hinduism for thousands of years. Meditation has also had a place in Judeo-Christian and Islamic cultures, as well as those of Native American and Pacific islanders, among others.

Examples of spiritual or faith-based meditation practices include **Kabbalah**, a form of Jewish mysticism, and **centering Christian prayer**. The latter involves the invocation of a sacred word and can include a movement meditation such as contemplative walking. Eastern examples of spiritual meditation include schools of Buddhist meditation that explore enlightenment and a path toward bliss, or Nirvana.

Movement Meditation

Some types of meditation feature some form of movement, often as a way of calming and bringing focus to the restless energy of the body. Movement meditation practices include contemplative walking, tai chi, qi gong, and some types of yoga.

Tai chi involves slow, graceful, and gentle body movements that are centered by awareness and focused, relaxed breathing. Tai chi, also known as movement meditation, grew out of an ancient form of martial arts practiced in China. Today, tai chi is used by seniors as well as by youth. While tai chi can be practiced alone, it is commonly practiced in groups.

The movements in tai chi—which one does while focusing on posture and breathing—are slow and flowing, one into the next, as though in slow motion. Concentration is maintained as intrusive thoughts are cast aside. This push-pull slow dance of opposite forces, the yin and yang of life in Chinese belief systems, fosters a greater flow of internal energy—what the Chinese call *qi*.

Many studies have pointed to the benefits of tai chi, especially for older adults. These benefits include improvements in physical as well as mental balance, bone mineral density, immune function, physical conditioning, cardiovascular fitness, and overall well-being. Some reports have described benefits for people who suffer from joint pain or osteoarthritis. The social and open-air practice of tai chi may also confer a sense of belonging, relaxation, and acceptance, as well as a connection with nature and the environment. For older adults, the added benefit of social and spiritual connectedness can also contribute to successful aging.

While tai chi typically involves a series of many small movements, another ancient Chinese practice, qi gong, involves doing the same movement many times. Whereas tai chi can include different postures and poses that require certain placement of the hands or feet, qi gong can be more suitable for people with limitations or those who prefer to begin a movement meditation more slowly or assuredly.

Learning Meditation

One size certainly does not fit all when it comes to meditation. Interested learners can choose from less-structured large-group settings or be guided by an instructor, whether in person or online, in small groups, or one-on-one. Many beginners find it comfortable to begin to learn how to meditate in the privacy of a quiet room at home. No matter what your personal preference, you can readily find tools, videos, MP3s, apps, courses, and books to help you learn to meditate (see the list of resources at the end of this chapter for more information).

Getting Started with Meditation: The Basics

The ability to meditate doesn't require a certain level of physical conditioning or fancy equipment. Here's what you'll need:

- A time of day that works for you (many meditators prefer mornings)
- An ambiance and room temperature that is comfortable for you
- A pillow, cushion, mat, or chair
- Loose, comfortable clothing
- As few distractions as possible

The process of meditating can take many forms. These nine steps will get you started:

1. Adjust to a comfortable seated pose; you may be most comfortable lying down.
2. Maintain a good posture: an upright spine and shoulders comfortably back.
3. Rest your hands on your lap or knees.
4. Keep your eyes open, and maintain soft focus on your surroundings. Or, find a point of focus such as the tip or bridge of your nose or a soft light.
5. Take slow breaths and experience the full length of each breath.
6. Focus on how the breath feels as it travels in and out of your body.
7. As thoughts enter your mind, acknowledge them, make no judgments about them, let them go, and refocus on the breath.
8. As you return focus and begin to enter a meditative state, feel your body in your mind, beginning with your feet and working upward.
9. Acknowledge your peace and feel gratitude for the experience.

Mindfulness programs or introductory meditation programs have sprouted up around the country, many of which include sessions that are tailored to the workplace or presented through a health facility. Larger towns and cities have established centers for various meditative approaches, such as Zen centers. Look for independent or community- or faith-based offerings in your vicinity.

Modern Mindfulness

In 1979, Jon Kabat-Zinn founded the Stress Reduction Clinic at the University of Massachusetts Medical School in Amherst. With a doctorate in molecular biology, Dr. Kabat-Zinn became interested in Zen teachings, Buddhism, and the potential of mindfulness in chronic disease states. A renowned educator and speaker, Kabat-Zinn has reached millions of people following his appearances on television and his many books (*Full Catastrophe Living*, 1991). His early center has grown into the Center for Mindfulness and offers a range of training and learning opportunities. The energy and work of Kabat-Zinn and his colleagues have not only helped bring mindfulness into the public eye but also have fostered mainstream acceptance and the study of meditation's many benefits.

Might You Benefit from Meditation and Other Mind-Body Therapies?

Meditation offers benefits for the mind, body, and spirit. Meditation and other mind-body therapies can be especially beneficial for individuals whose lives are often affected or disrupted by any of the following:

- Very stressful situations on a routine basis
- Feeling a lack of control
- A sense of unpredictability or uncertainty about life or the future
- The inability to maintain focus or to follow through
- Difficulty in setting goals or reaching reasonable targets
- Excessive distractibility or mind wandering
- Repetitive negative thoughts that are not associated with a goal
- Excessive worry
- Feeling caught in a cycle of stress-distress–more stress
- A tendency to view situations or individuals as insurmountable, threats, or anxiety-provoking rather than as challenges

Uses and Evidence for Meditation

Remember that meditation is a practice, and the practice it requires may be lengthy or frustrating for some people. Unlike other forms of healing, meditation may not be a quick fix. Instructors and settings vary, and some may not be to your liking. Without a recognized national meditation society, it can require some research and legwork to find a meditation setting that works for you. Keep an open mind, and discuss your interest in meditation with your health-care team.

Once you get better at meditation, you'll find the practice quite portable and handy. The ability to meditate is something you can learn to carry inside yourself—to rediscover and experience wherever you may be. Consider the different types of meditation to find a style that suits your needs and lifestyle.

Below are some of the common uses of meditation, many of which are listed alongside other therapies and methods in Chapter 14. Evidence of effectiveness is stronger for those conditions starred with an asterisk (*).

Useful in:

- Anxiety*
- Depression*
- Pain*
- High blood pressure*
- Heart/blood vessel diseases*
- Cancer supportive care

Also used in/for:

- Stress*
- Sleep disorders
- Substance abuse
- Attention deficits
- Menopausal symptoms
- Irritable bowel syndrome

Uncertain or not helpful in/for:

- Weight control
- More severe psychiatric conditions

Is Meditation Safe?

Overall, meditation and mind-body therapies are safe treatments in most people. Although few studies have reported on specific or potential harmful effects of meditation, studies that looked at major systems of the body found no significant harmful effects of meditation.

Because the benefits of meditation for conditions such as high blood pressure may be more variable or less dramatic than the effects triggered by medications and other interventions, it's important to share this information with your health-care team. Together you can decide whether the benefit gained from this or any other practice is enough on its own or whether you may also need to explore other ways to help bring down and maintain your blood pressure at a safe and sustainable level.

You may also want to discuss with your care team certain movement meditation practices that interest you, particularly the more physically challenging practices like Bikram yoga, which is discussed below. Some movement meditations may present challenges if you are at high risk for fractures or balance problems. Engage your health-care team to work with you to offer guidance that will allow you to pursue beneficial mind-body interventions in a safe, effective way.

YOGA

Yoga is a mind-body practice rooted in ancient Indian philosophy, traditions, and Hinduism. Believed to bring about harmony of mind, body, and spirit, yoga also is said to unite the consciousness of the individual with that of the cosmos. Yoga requires patience, discipline, and practice to achieve the benefits that make yoga so useful and appealing in health and wellness.

Yoga involves breathing methods, meditation, positions, and stretches that are believed to trigger or interact with different internal pathways, leading to the desired effects of calm; a sense of wellness; and perhaps the easing of pain, anxiety, or other troublesome conditions.

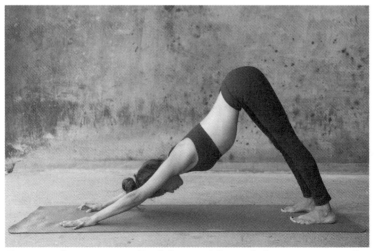

Yoga can bring greater flexibility and better balance, among other benefits.

Yoga Styles

The most popular form of yoga in the U.S. is **hatha** yoga, which focuses on breathing (pranayama), meditation, and poses or postures called **asanas**. The varied yoga methods focus on aligning the energy centers of the body or vortices, known as **chakras**.

There are many yoga styles from which to choose. Some styles include chanting, while others do not. From the vigorous to the more relaxing types, yoga styles can accommodate a wide variety of fitness levels, ages, and physical needs or limitations.

Common Yoga Types

Type	Description
Ashtanga	An intense, physical style with a specific set and order of poses; the basis of power yoga in the U.S.
Bikram	A sequence of hatha poses in a sauna-like heated studio.
Iyengar	Follows the instructor's lead with props and poses held for long periods of time.
Kripalu	Deep meditation with movement and postures.
Vinyasa	Step-by-step flowing progression with rhythmic breathing.

Yoga is one of the most popular, approachable, and nontoxic mind-body methods. In the U.S., the use of yoga has steadily climbed in national health surveys taken in 2002, 2007, and 2012. Over the past decade, yoga has been increasingly studied, producing a great deal of information about its benefits. Besides enhancing wellness, fitness, and quality of life, yoga has also been shown to aid the following conditions:

- Lower back pain
- Anxiety
- Pain
- Depression
- High blood pressure
- Insomnia
- Fibromyalgia

Some evidence also indicates that yoga may also be helpful for certain types of arthritis, eating disorders, headaches, cancer-related fatigue, post-traumatic stress disorder, and menopausal symptoms. Although yoga appears to improve lung function in healthy people, the evidence for yoga in asthma appears ambiguous.

Is Yoga for Everyone?

Interest in yoga continues to surge. Today, yoga is one of the top ten integrative health approaches. While most people could benefit from yoga, certain individuals should talk about their interest in yoga with their health provider before embarking on a yoga path that could be too strenuous or possibly harmful to their health.

For example, people with heart or breathing problems or high blood pressure should be especially cautious with the more fast-paced or physically demanding forms of yoga, especially hot yoga or Bikram. The same goes for people taking multiple medications and those with weak bones, with glaucoma, or at risk for blood clots. Women who are pregnant or nursing may wish to limit themselves to the gentler forms of yoga, which can deliver similar benefits, until after childbirth or breast-feeding.

How to Find a Yoga Instructor

Because yoga is not a regulated practice, individuals may identify themselves as yoga instructors without being sufficiently trained, competent, or committed to ethical practice. Ask trusted health-care providers or friends with experience with a trained and certified yoga instructor for a recommendation. Another source is the International Association of Yoga Therapists, which is developing a credentialing program for yoga instructors. Some members of the National Ayurvedic Medical Association are also yoga teachers.

BIOFEEDBACK

Biofeedback uses the replay or feedback of information such as pulse rate or skin temperature gathered through the use of special devices or monitoring equipment to help the client harness the power of the mind to influence those functions toward more positive outcomes.

For example, a person with high blood pressure may observe through monitoring that their breaths are short and shallow or that their heart rate slows and speeds up in an irregular way. By reading the cues provided by the devices, such individuals can be trained to breathe slower and deeper, to use other powers of focus and concentration to steady their heart rate, to release their muscle tension, or to use another relaxation mode to help bring down their blood pressure or steady their rhythm.

After relaxation techniques have been learned in the high-tech setting of monitors and with the guidance of a biofeedback therapist, successful users of biofeedback eventually are able to summon their relaxation response from within—without the need for devices or perhaps the instructor—whether to help control headaches, blood pressure, or anxiety, or for any of the other uses of biofeedback.

A typical biofeedback session lasts for 30 to 60 minutes. First, the therapist will apply one or more painless monitoring devices to your scalp, skin, or other areas. Then, the information gathered through such monitoring will be shared with you using sounds or other means. Once you have learned to associate the monitored functions of your body with the cue, you can begin to learn to use your mental powers, relaxation exercises, breathing, and any coaching involved to alter those functions more positively.

During the process, you can realize a new level of control as you learn to become your own monitor, interpreting and modifying your body's responses through the cues you are given and the relaxation techniques learned.

Despite being technology-driven at the onset, biofeedback is an otherwise natural, nontoxic way to reverse the "fight or flight" response or to turn off noxious and negative thought processes that can work against health and wellness.

However, akin to massage therapy, the success of biofeedback treatment depends in large part on the skill of the operator, or therapist. Many university programs have skilled biofeedback therapists on staff or will know of reliable practitioners you may wish to consult.

Uses of Biofeedback

Biofeedback has been successfully used to help treat headaches in children, adult tension headaches, high blood pressure, anxiety, and different types of pain—including that due to fibromyalgia, temporomandibular joint disorders, and rheumatoid arthritis. Biofeedback training has also been useful in stroke recovery and constipation, and it appears to help people with some types of incontinence.

Other conditions for which biofeedback is being studied and may be useful include ringing in the ears (tinnitus), attention deficit hyperactivity disorder (ADHD), and smoking cessation, among others.

How to Find a Biofeedback Practitioner

Biofeedback practitioners may be located at *aapb.org*. The Biofeedback Certification Alliance offers board certification in different areas of biofeedback along with ethics requirements that are recognized by national and international biofeedback organizations.

HYPNOTHERAPY

Hypnosis or hypnotherapy is a deep form of relaxation therapy that can be achieved on your own with training, with the help of an app (self-hypnosis), or with the aid of a hypnotherapist. To achieve this deep state of relaxation, a trained therapist offers suggestions and guidance, often by repeating certain words or cues to help bring you into and out of a hypnotic state. Once you have been hypnotized into a trance-like state, you are able to hold deep focus and feel centered by calm and tranquility.

There are several uses of hypnotherapy, many of which are similar to those for guided imagery. Hypnotherapy can help with anxiety relief or can work as an aid to help you achieve a better sense of control so that you can better pursue or reach your goals. Hypnotherapy is also used to help remove obstacles blocking behavior change that is needed or wanted for better health. Hypnosis can help to relieve stress related to an upcoming procedure or event, such as before surgery, a dental procedure, or cancer treatments.

Uses of Hypnotherapy

Hypnotherapy is commonly used as an integrative practice for irritable bowel syndrome (IBS). Such therapy may help IBS patients better manage not only IBS-specific symptoms but also the anxiety and depression that sometimes accompany the disease or bouts of disease activity. Such relief typically leads to better overall functioning and improved quality of life.

Pain is another common symptom that may be helped by hypnosis. Studies have shown promising results for pain related to arthritis as well as fibromyalgia, temporomandibular joint pain, pain related to cancer or its treatment, and headaches. Hypnosis can also help with the nausea brought on by the anticipation of chemotherapy.

Hot flashes, whether related to menopause or those that occur as a result of certain therapies for breast cancer, also appear to be aided by hypnotherapy.

Behavioral issues for which hypnotherapy could be helpful include smoking cessation and weight control in obese individuals. Hypnosis has also been used successfully for simple phobias and habitual coughing or coughing that does not appear to have a lung-related or other physical component.

In children, hypnotherapy offers a drug-free, nontoxic option that has been used successfully for bed wetting and holds promise for childhood functional abdominal pain disorders, anxiety, and other behavioral troubles.

Hypnotherapy does not appear to be useful for inducing labor in pregnant women. In addition, because attempting hypnosis may delay much-needed care, its use in this setting cannot be recommended in general. However, exceptions are possible, perhaps in special circumstances involving highly trained personnel, nearby obstetrical facilities, and patients who have been adequately prepared for such an intervention.

Side Effects and Cautions

Hypnotherapy is generally a well-tolerated and nontoxic therapy when guided by a competent therapist. The chances of having a successful result from hypnosis appear partly related to how open-minded or receptive you are to the idea of being hypnotized.

However, because hypnosis may bring on powerful emotions, hypnosis may paradoxically increase distress or anxiety in some people. Headaches have also been reported. Also, the remembrances that may be called up or explored in a hypnosis session may be distorted—perhaps even deceiving or disturbing.

How to Find a Hypnotherapist

Hypnotherapy is a diverse field, representing many types of professionals—from chiropractors, dentists, and medical doctors to licensed family therapists, social workers, and different types of counselors. Find an experienced, certified, and credentialed practitioner using the links at the end of this chapter.

GUIDED IMAGERY

Guided imagery is a healing tool that uses the power, emotions, and memories associated with a mental image (visualization) to reach a desired goal. In connecting the mind and body, the goals of guided imagery can vary from person to person.

Such goals may be related to influencing your heart rate, blood pressure, or anxiety level; gaining greater insight regarding your behaviors; finding hope or motivation to make a life change; or finding calm to nurture your spirit.

Visualization techniques are an old tradition. They have been used in various care systems to spur healing or to promote vitality. The ancient Greeks and Navajo tribes used imagery techniques, which are also used in traditional Chinese medicine. Beyond its many uses in healing, guided imagery has also been used in the modern era to enhance sports performance or achievement, notably in golf and tennis.

Most of us typically use imagery regularly in other ways, sometimes negatively. We commonly use our imagination and mental images for problem solving and challenges, as in worrying about and visualizing the many things that might go wrong during a decision-making process. We also use imagery that is imbued with optimism or to plan for the future, as when we decorate a dream house in our mind or imagine what we would do or want to do if we won the lottery.

Until recently, however, imagery was not typically used by most people to connect with its full healing potential, or to help them envision and connect with a change in health behaviors.

Yet, there is good evidence that practicing guided imagery can bring relaxation and healthful benefits in many settings. Some evidence even suggests that guided imagery can help increase the number of helpful immune cells. Small studies in women with breast cancer have found that guided imagery, sometimes with another form of relaxation therapy, improved cancer patients' quality of life and emotional balance.

Guided imagery also can be helpful for the anxiety faced before surgery or before a procedure, as in cancer care, and for other stresses of daily living. Guided imagery may also be helpful in stroke rehabilitation and in recovery from trauma, as with nightmares that may occur in post-traumatic stress disorder.

Learning Guided Imagery: One-on-One, Small Groups, Books, Apps, or DVDs

Many options are available to learn guided imagery. Books, apps, or DVDs can be used to learn the techniques on your own, or you can learn interactively with a therapist or in a small group. Soft and calming music is usually played as you learn how to follow the steps of the method, beginning with physical relaxation and mental focus with calm breathing. Then, you are coached to visualize an image that makes you feel safe, calm, and comfortable. The therapist or DVD may offer other suggestions to help you develop the image and positive associations with it in your mind. Therapists also guide you toward focus and refocus as needed along the way.

The final phase in guided imagery is called affirmation, in which you learn to associate the now-familiar mental image that you have learned to call up with the positive messaging and the goals associated with it.

Uses of Guided Imagery

Besides stress and anxiety, guided imagery can also be helpful in cancer care or in managing other chronic illnesses, including headaches. The positivity and sense of control that are stimulated by affirmations may also be helpful for smoking cessation and other types of substance abuse.

Another area where guided imagery may help bring calm and perhaps solace is in end-of-life care. Guided imagery can also be used as a motivational tool to aid people in making lifestyle changes or during difficult transition periods in life that may require change or major adjustments. Examples include profound grief after a loss or familial, work, or marital conflicts. Some practitioners are finding success combining guided imagery with massage or another touch therapy.

Finding a Guided Imagery Practitioner

Professionally certified guided imagery practitioners include counselors, doctors, nurses, therapists, and other health-care professionals. Go to *acadgi.com* to find a trained and certified practitioner.

OTHER THERAPIES AND BIOENERGETICS

Music Therapy

Music is emotional. Music can evoke positive feelings that are rousing, soothing, or inspiring. The ancient Greek philosopher Plato was said to observe that music is what gives the universe a soul, provides the mind its wings to soar, gives flight to the imagination, and brings joy and charm to life and all else.

Today, in health and wellness, music is being used as a type of mind-body therapy to bring calm and to help relieve symptoms such as those related to stress, pain, and other conditions. The beauty, familiarity, and rhythm of music has been particularly useful and promising for the agitation associated with earlier forms of Alzheimer's disease, for some psychiatric conditions (including depression), and to promote greater quality of life and well-being in end-of-life care. Music therapy has also been used to foster progress and encouragement during rehabilitation, as in after major surgery or with debilitation or stroke.

Anesthesiologists have used a type of music therapy for decades to help patients awaiting surgery feel less anxious and more comfortable in the cold, unfamiliar, and sterile surroundings of the surgical suite.

Nontoxic and pleasant, music therapy can be helpful for different mood disorders and—in hospitalized patients or people with serious conditions—can aid in coping, disease management, and pain or stress reduction. Even in the high-tech environment of intensive care units, patients receiving music therapy have been shown to have less anxiety and to require fewer and less frequent sedatives.

Early studies have also been encouraging regarding the use of music therapy to help restore brain function and emotional adjustment after traumatic brain injury.

Trained music therapists assess each individual patient to determine his or her needs and the goals of therapy. Depending on the need, the choice of music or activity may be aimed at fostering tranquility, emotional intimacy, social interaction, or stimulation or a better sense of control. A therapist may choose to engage the patient by playing selected music or may have the patient participate in a music activity, one-on-one or in groups. Advanced music therapy may also include music songwriting or the noncompetitive playing of an instrument.

Being emotional in nature, music therapy can also help foster connectedness between the care team and the patient and his or her family, or within families, while also providing relaxation and pleasure.

Although encouraging, the long-term effects and effectiveness of music therapy are largely unexplored. Yet, in the short term, it is an inexpensive and nontoxic stimulus that appears to offer calm and centering for certain situations and individuals.

Aromatherapy

In aromatherapy, the aromas released by essential oils are used to calm, stimulate, or bring balance to an individual.

The aromatic oils may be applied onto the skin by compresses or through massage. Alternatively, the oils can be inhaled using a diffuser, steam or sprays, or with an aroma lamp. Full-body aroma baths can be chosen, or only the feet or hands may be immersed in aroma-enhanced waters. Taking aromatic oils internally, whether rectally or by mouth, can be toxic or harmful and is not recommended.

Lavender and lemon are two of the most common essential oils used in aromatherapy. Although people who use aromatherapy report feeling better with regard to stress, anxiety, depression, some pain, sleep disorders, and other conditions, the evidence for the effectiveness of aromatherapy—especially beyond the short-term—remains weak. Despite claims to the contrary, aromatherapy has not proved useful for immunity. However, nontoxic therapies such as this may be considered as part of an integrative care plan alongside other therapies that have greater and more reliable effectiveness.

Read more about aromatherapy and essential oils in Chapter 9.

Reiki

Reiki was developed in Japan in the early 1900s, reaching the U.S. mainland in the 1940s following its introduction to Hawaii. A touch method of energy healing, Reiki takes its name from the Japanese word for universal energy (rei) and ki, similar to the meaning of the Chinese word qi, signifying the bioenergy within living creatures.

Trained Reiki practitioners use their hands, either just above the clothed client or atop the skin, with the goal of rebalancing or restoring the recipient's energy flow to allow the body to heal. Reiki is used for overall well-being and as a restorative relaxation or healing therapy.

Although Reiki has been used in a variety of settings, including in patients undergoing hospital care as well as less acute conditions such as chronic pain and stress-related disorders, the evidence for the effectiveness of Reiki remains weak. However, because Reiki is nontoxic in itself and may benefit people in need of stress relief or distress from illness, Reiki is gaining more widespread adoption that may lead to better trials and more convincing evidence.

Hospitals are beginning to offer Reiki therapy, and some are experimenting with Reiki training for caregivers or family of pediatric, cancer, and other types of patients. The hope is that such training and practice may provide some degree of control and comfort for both the patients and their families as they cope with illness or the effects of difficult therapies.

Training and certification of Reiki practitioners is not standardized. Different levels of training may be achieved. Holistic nurses and other trained health-care professionals have shown interest in gaining Reiki training and experience. Look for professionals who have embraced ethical standards in their corresponding fields of expertise.

Healing Touch Therapies

In this type of bioenergetics therapy, practitioners use their hands above and then gently on the body, aiming to assess and then to realign the client's energy fields for healing and restoration. Healing touch is rooted in many different ancient cultures and is used therapeutically with other cultural or spiritual beliefs or practices.

The uses of healing touch are similar to those for Reiki. Like Reiki, the evidence of effectiveness is spotty and mostly anecdotal. Some studies have combined the effects of touch and no-touch methods, which makes the results difficult to interpret.

Clients who have experienced these types of **biofield** therapies frequently report feeling a greater sense of stress relief, relaxation, or a restoration of well-being. The science behind these therapies and their true utility, however, remain incompletely understood.

Magnet Therapy

The mysterious power of magnetic attraction has captured the imagination of children and healers for centuries. Historically, magnets have been used to treat a range of conditions and ailments, from baldness to poisoning.

The basic belief of magnetic healing is that magnetic forces, whether generated by a magnetic field or by using actual static magnets, can foster healing.

Like other types of biofield beliefs that are gaining traction among the public, notably with types of energy that cannot be seen, magnet therapy also has its debunkers. Theories about simple magnets' abilities to transform or realign cells or certain cellular functions have not passed scientific muster.

Nonetheless, a few experiments have suggested some degree of benefit for magnetic field therapies using electromagnets, unlike the static type of magnet you might have played with as a child.

Electromagnetic field therapy has shown promise in speeding up fracture healing, notably in fractures that are not mending together as a result of standard care, known as nonunion fractures. Other conditions that have been resistant to other treatments and that might benefit from electromagnetic field therapy include arthritis, depression, and fibromyalgia. Another study reported success in treating people with insomnia using low-energy emission therapy, a type of electromagnetic therapy that was administered inside the mouth.

Preliminary studies in animals are exploring whether electromagnetic fields can halt the growth or spread of tumor cells when used in conjunction with other methods such as radiation. In humans, promising early results have been obtained with a particularly lethal form of brain cancer. However, many of these studies have been funded by companies or conducted by investigators involved in the magnetism device industry. Results from unbiased studies will help clarify the debate.

Static magnet therapy has received attention for many diseases, notably arthritis (osteoarthritis, the more common type), chronic pain, and other musculoskeletal problems. Among these popular items are magnets you can wear in your shoes or add to your bedding, or magnetic bracelets or bands that wrap around the wrist or knee. Notwithstanding the testimonials in ads and on television, scientific evidence for the effectiveness of these types of devices has not been demonstrated.

Know that the use of magnets can interfere with implanted devices such as pacemakers or insulin pumps. Reconsider the use of magnets when other proven and effective methods are available.

If you are interested in magnet therapy or any other therapy for which the benefits are in doubt or are still being evaluated, consider enrolling in a clinical trial. Search for trials on a variety of treatments and for an array of conditions at *www.clinicaltrials.gov*.

WHERE TO LEARN MORE

University of Massachusetts Worchester Campus Center for Mindfulness: *http://www.umassmed.edu/cfm/*

Transcendental meditation: *www.tm.org, www.tm-meditation.co.uk*

The Relaxation Response by Herbert Benson, M.D.: Updated (2009) version of the groundbreaking book originally published in 1975

International Association of Yoga Therapists: *www.iayt.org*

National Ayurvedic Medical Association: *www.ayurvedanama.org*

Association for Applied Psychophysiology and Biofeedback: *www.aapb.org*

Academy for Guided Imagery: *www.acadgi.com*

American Society of Clinical Hypnosis: *www.asch.net*

American Music Therapy Association: *www.musictherapy.org*

8

Manual Therapies and Bodywork

ODYWORK INCLUDES A HOST OF STYLES AND TYPES OF MANUAL THERAPIES. As a laying-on of hands, manual bodywork can be not only relaxing and soothing but also therapeutic for various ailments and conditions.

Common examples of bodywork include a variety of massage techniques; reflexology; osteopathic or chiropractic manipulation; and special methods such as Rolfing, Feldenkrais, or Alexander that are described in this chapter. Other common names for this area of practice or study are manual medicine or therapeutic massage and bodywork.

The general category of massage includes a wide range of techniques, some of which are gentle and slow. Others involve more forceful, deep, or rapid movements. Deciding which type of bodywork is right for you can depend on your physical comfort level, state of health, preference for a clothed or unclothed experience, or perhaps your receptiveness to physical touch itself.

Certain types of bodywork are more passive than others, requiring the therapist or bodyworker to perform the work as the patient or client experiences the treatment. Other methods such as the Alexander or Feldenkrais techniques entail having the patient or client participate more actively in the session, as with learning to retrain their body awareness, habits, and posture.

Individuals who prefer to remain clothed may find techniques such as reflexology more suitable to their needs, whereas individuals seeking or in need of deep tissue stimulation may prefer Rolfing. In addition, some bodywork practices are sometimes performed in groups, while others are best experienced during one-on-one contact.

This chapter aims to help you decide which manual therapy will meet your needs.

THE HEALING POWER OF TOUCH

Although it seems logical or intuitive that touch therapy, whether through massage or other manipulative techniques, would provide positive health benefits, one wonders: is there a scientific basis for the healing power of touch?

As it turns out, many benefits of touch therapies have been supported by scientific studies. Massage, being one of the most frequently studied, increases blood flow to the stimulated tissues, partly because massage warms the massaged area. Massage also loosens or eases muscle tension, which in turn also helps calm overly excited nerve pathways that can trigger pain or persistent muscle tightness.

On a deeper level, massage can stimulate certain reflexes that lead to a lowering of the heart rate and blood pressure. Another way that massage may elicit a calming response or a sense of well-being is through hormones and the body's internal chemicals. Massage appears to help dial back stimulating hormones such as cortisol and vasopressin. Massage can also ramp up levels of oxytocin, dubbed the "love hormone" for its association with bonding behaviors such as that between mothers and their newborns or that associated with affectionate behaviors such as hugging and kissing.

On another level, massage can also increase levels of nitrous oxide, an important chemical made in our bodies that helps blood vessels relax. Massage can also stimulate the production of beta-endorphins, our inner analgesic that is also released with exercise.

BODYWORK: USES AND EFFECTIVENESS

The usefulness of manual medicine has been recognized for thousands of years. Massage was used in traditional healing by the ancient Chinese and in Ayurveda using warm oils. Famously championed by the ancient Greeks and Romans, massage was prescribed for sprains and other conditions by Hippocrates and later by Galen.

Although bodywork can be useful by itself, manual therapies are often at their best when they are integrated into a whole-person approach to care. Take the common example of neck pain, a condition that has been estimated to affect 15% of adults at some time. Massage has been shown to be a useful, drug-free method that provides symptom relief. Even though the relief from weekly or twice-weekly massage therapy might not reach 100%, the amount of symptom relief can still be enough to improve a neck pain sufferer's quality of life and daily functioning. Also, regular massage for neck pain may also provide a pain-free window during which the neck pain is eased to a degree that allows the sufferer to use less pain medication or to resume certain activities.

The Birth of Modern Massage

Although massage today is not considered a form of exercise or gymnastics, the roots of modern massage and physical therapy can be traced to Pehr Henrik Ling, who founded Sweden's Central Royal Gymnastic Institute in 1813. Ling observed that kneading, pressing, and rubbing seemed to alleviate his own health ailments and called these movements "medical gymnastics." His findings led him first to study and then to teach the benefits of manipulation, which became known as the Swedish Movement Cure. Later in the 1800s, the Dutch practitioner Johan Georg Mezger developed a way to categorize the various massage methods being used, codifying these techniques using French words such as *effleurage* (a fingertip-light and gliding stroke) and *frictions* (a deeper rubbing). The writings and influence of these two pioneers garnered the attention of doctors and other health practitioners of the day, giving rise to the classical Western massage style of long, gliding strokes that came to be known as Swedish massage.

A Medicare study that looked at overall health-care costs found that users of CAM for neck and back pain, including massage therapy, were associated with lower overall costs than non-CAM users, suggesting that the successful use of integrative approaches for these conditions can also be cost-saving or cost-effective.

The success of manual therapies may vary widely depending on the technique used, the suitability of the method used to the patient's needs, the individual skill of the provider, the frequency of its use or the session length, and the setting, among other factors. Because of this variability, many trials that have attempted to test the effectiveness of massage versus other less variable treatments, such as a prescription drug, have been flawed or incomplete. Nevertheless, many good studies continue to emerge.

These are a few of the general conditions for which massage has been shown to be helpful, at least temporarily, along with specific examples for which the evidence is strongest:

- Chronic pain (lower back, neck)
- Muscle soreness (related to sports, activity)
- Arthritis (osteoarthritis of the knee)

- Cancer (for pain and relaxation and to improve mood, anxiety, and fatigue)
- Depression (in pregnant women)
- Anxiety (various conditions, including smoking cessation)
- Headache (chronic tension headaches)
- Fibromyalgia
- HIV/AIDS (in regard to quality of life)
- Infant care (pre-term infant weight gain)

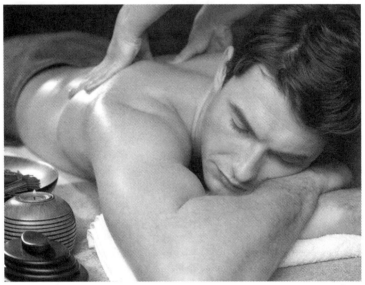

Back massage involves rubbing and manipulating muscles and soft tissues.

Massage also appears to be helpful with the pain of labor, migraines, and some types of depression as well as for behavioral issues such as autism. Foot massage may also be helpful for dementia-associated agitation.

Surgery is another area where massage has been shown to help relieve pain and anxiety associated with procedures and cardiac care. Promising work has also pointed to possible immune function benefits in women with breast cancer and in HIV care, although these studies have not reported improved survival or outcomes to date.

Other conditions for which massage may offer at least temporary relief of symptoms include the movement difficulties in Parkinson's disease, insomnia, and spasticity problems in amyotrophic lateral sclerosis (ALS). Belly massage can also be helpful for chronic constipation, a condition that deserves a full evaluation before relying solely on massage for relief.

MANUAL METHODS: SAFETY PROFILE

In general, massage and other manual therapies have an excellent safety profile—that is, the complication rate is low and the rate of serious or life-threatening complications is extremely low.

Like all therapies, however, problems can occur. The most common complaint after manual therapies relates to muscle soreness, although this is usually minor and typically will resolve on its own within a day or two.

More serious complications have been reported, although they are rare. A review that looked at reports in all languages of manipulative therapy- and massage-related complications in world literature from 2003 to 2013 found that disc herniation was the most common reported complication, followed by trauma to the soft tissues (muscle and skin), nerves, and blood vessels; spinal cord injury; and fracture and bleeding, among others. Most (60%) of the adverse reports came from China. Of all the complications compiled, only about 6% involved various types of massage therapists. Nearly a quarter of the overall complications involved chiropractors. Practitioners whose professional status was unknown or who were said to be unregistered were involved in the majority of the reported problems.

The safety of chiropractic manipulation is discussed further in Chapter 10.

Getting Rubbed the Right Way: Safety and Comfort

In most cases, massage is a nontoxic, drug-free, and safe practice. You can take an active role in keeping yourself out of harm's way by letting your therapist know of any underlying conditions or problems you are having that might be worsened or could be risky with manual manipulation.

Share the following information with both the practitioner who recommends manual therapy to you as well as the therapist or bodyworker before your session:

- Any history of bleeding problems or tendencies
- Any medications you are taking, especially those that interfere with bleeding (blood thinners); those that relate to a heart condition or high blood pressure and those taken for any psychiatric or balance disturbances, including herbal remedies
- Any history or risk for stroke or clotting disorders (including previous blood clots in your legs or lungs or associated with pregnancy or hormones)

- Any recent surgery, orthopedic problems, burns, or an area of your body that is healing (even if the overlying skin has healed)
- Whether you might have osteoporosis or weak or brittle bones
- Any history of cancer, bone tumors or radiation therapy
- Heart or nerve conditions you may have, including any conditions that cause you to have light-headedness or seizures
- Any sore spots that might be too tender for direct pressure
- Implants, devices, or surgery you have had

Your own personal comfort is another high-priority item, in terms of both your physical and psychological comfort levels.

Certain massage or manipulation methods do not require that you fully or partially disrobe. Reflexology is applied to the foot, and certain styles of massage such as anma, or traditional Japanese massage, are done through clothing without the use of lubricants. Loose clothing or a gown can be worn for many osteopathic or chiropractic manipulations, too.

Besides clothing or modesty concerns, communicate with your therapist about your preferences. Seemingly mundane issues such as whether the therapy room is too hot or too cold for you can influence feelings of success or satisfaction with your session. Being physically comfortable may also influence your willingness to continue with your sessions or to pursue the therapy period through to the goal.

Let your therapist know if the pressure level is too light or too deep, or whether or not you prefer to engage in conversation during your session. Sound is important, too. Music that may be soothing to one client might be intrusive to a person who wants a more peaceful, silent experience. Remember that your therapist aims to provide a good outcome for you and that you will both benefit from your feedback. Bodyworkers want and need your input; let them know how you feel and what you hope to gain at any time before, during, or after your session.

Manual therapies are designed to provide an uplifting experience, whether through stimulation, release, relaxation, or relief of troublesome symptoms. Partner with your therapist and health-care team to help create your best possible experience.

TRAINING AND LICENSURE

Massage has soared in popularity among Americans. In a one-year period from 2012 to 2013, an estimated 35 million Americans, or 16% of the population, experienced at least one massage, according to statistics compiled by the American Massage Therapy Association and the U.S. government. Among this group, 43% reported that the massage was intended as therapy for a health or medical condition, such as pain, spasm, and recovery from an injury, or for wellness.

With more than 300,000 massage therapists and students nationwide, massage therapist employment in the U.S. is expected to grow 20% between 2010 and 2020, according to U.S. Department of Labor statistics. What's more, these statistics may only include a fraction of the bodyworkers who specialize in one of the estimated 250 types of bodywork. Clearly, interest in manual medicine is on the rise.

So how can a health-care consumer know that the person from whom they are seeking care is adequately trained? Or whether or not their practice is guided by a strict code of ethics to which they have pledged? Or, just as important, one must ask if the practitioner has been certified by a reputable organization and is licensed to practice that method according to his or her state's regulations.

As of 2014, 44 states and the District of Columbia either provided a voluntary method of certification or had regulations on record for massage therapy practitioners. These regulations typically include a certain minimum number of hours of training that bodyworkers must undergo and/or passing a licensing exam.

Licensed massage therapists can be expected to have graduated from one of the more than 360 accredited programs in the U.S., where they receive an average of nearly 650 hours of training, according to the American Massage Therapy Association. Additionally, most practicing massage therapists participate in continuing education to stay abreast of new knowledge and techniques, as well as to refine or expand their skills.

Be sure to ask whether the practitioner you will see is state licensed and whether he or she completed training at an accredited massage therapy school. Also ask whether the therapist is a member of the American Massage Therapy Association or the Association of Bodywork & Massage Professionals (ABMP). In addition to massage therapists, the ABMP also includes practices beyond conventional massage therapy. Both organizations require members to adhere to codes of ethics.

The training and certification requirements for the many types of specialized bodywork practitioners are highly variable. Use the links at the end of this chapter to help guide you toward practitioners who have undergone special training and certification, who subscribe to ethical practices, and who are licensed. Be wary of practices that seem geared toward purchases of more services or expensive products that you do not need.

MANUAL THERAPIES: DIFFERENT STROKES

If you are pursuing bodywork on your own, begin by examining whether a particular type of bodywork suits your preference and goals. Some therapies are more passive, active, softer, or firmer. Certain types such as acupressure have a component of energy healing, while other manual therapies integrate guided imagery, aromatherapy, or music therapy with the manual arts.

Some of these services may be covered in part by your health insurance, usually with a referral by your physician or a qualified health-care professional.

Peruse this section to find the massage style that suits your health goals and personal needs. Do you want clothing on or off? A soft, gliding touch or deep-tissue kneading? One of the many styles below will hopefully fulfill your needs.

Swedish Massage

Also called classical massage, this technique calls for a lighter to medium touch. It delivers smooth, long, and gliding strokes directed toward the heart, which is believed to foster better circulation and energy. This method can also include kneading, rolling, and other firmer manipulations on oiled or lubricated skin. Typically, the client fully or partially disrobes before the session and is covered by draping sheets or towels.

This type of massage may be useful for general relaxation, enhanced wellness, tightness, soreness or pain, and stress-related conditions.

Thai Massage

Based on a traditional belief that the body is composed of certain lines of energy, this type of massage stimulates outer parts of the body with the aim of stimulating inner parts to which they are believed to be connected by energy streams. The client usually remains clothed, except for footwear, and is positioned on a floor mat or mattress rather than a massage table. Therapists use their body weight to apply pressure, which can be done with hands, forearms, knees, and feet. Movements are firm and rhythmic, with deep compressions, pulls, and stretches aimed at enhancing energy and restoring balance. The client is sometimes positioned in twisted or yoga-like poses. Therapy can be received one-on-one or in small groups. Sometimes, breathing exercises are also taught and then performed. Traditional sessions can last for two hours or more, depending on the therapist and the client's needs.

This type of massage may be useful for enhanced mindfulness, osteoarthritis (knee), and myofascial pain.

Chinese Massage (Tui Na)

Also known as tui na, Chinese massage involves a variety of manual techniques ranging from pulling, squeezing, and shaking to pressing, stroking, and rubbing. Depending on the client's needs, tui na can be gentle but is typically more stimulating and vigorous. As with other Asian massage styles, it also seeks to restore energy flows, which are considered to improve body function and to strengthen the body against disease.

This type of massage may be useful for chronic pain or stiffness, high blood pressure (integrated with conventional care), and stress-related conditions.

Japanese Massage (Anwa or Amma)

This method follows an established sequence of movements applied to acupressure points along the body. Practitioners use their hands, knuckles, feet, and knees to press, tap, stretch, and rub, typically without using lubricants. Unlike Swedish massage, the movements are directed away from the heart. Clients may lie down or sit, making this method more accommodating for people with limited mobility or modesty concerns.

This type of massage may be useful for chronic pain or stiffness and movement disorders (Parkinson's).

Shiatsu

This is a Japanese technique derived from anma that uses tapping motions of the fingertips, palms, or usually the thumbs over traditional acupressure/acupuncture sites. Shiatsu is often practiced in a prescribed sequence or for set periods of time, with the goal of releasing or restoring energy and balance. Shiatsu is usually performed on a soft floor mat on a loosely clothed individual, but it can also involve rolling or rotation movements and stretching. Shiatsu, like other massage techniques, may be useful for general relaxation, enhanced wellness, tightness, soreness or pain, and stress-related conditions. Although it has been recommended for a variety of disturbances and ailments beyond these, there is little evidence to support many other uses.

Getting in Touch

Other types of bodywork you might consider for certain circumstances in life include deep tissue massage, lomi lomi, and watsu.

Deep tissue massage isn't simply a deeper version of the traditional Swedish massage and is best performed by trained practitioners. The bodyworker applies slower, deeper strokes that go against the grain of muscles, aiming to also stimulate connective tissues. This can be a useful technique for sport-related aches and pains.

Lomi lomi is a type of Hawaiian bodywork rooted in cultural beliefs related to wholeness, love, and nurturing. With its long and gliding strokes, this type of technique is worth considering to boost overall wellness, lessen anxiety, and heighten well-being and connectedness. Some practitioners use prayer or chanting in their sessions.

Watsu is a newer type of bodywork that brings together elements of shiatsu and water therapy. The bodyworker holds the client afloat in warm water, applying gentle stretches and shiatsu techniques along the body. Pregnant women may especially find this gentle, drug-free combination of massage and hydrotherapy to be relaxing and soothing.

REFLEXOLOGY

According to reflexology, certain areas of the feet, hands, and ears are believed to have a connection or "reflex" with deeper areas of the body. In line with this belief, the proper stimulation of these external points is considered to trigger far-reaching effects on deeper organs or inner body systems.

When performed by a trained practitioner, supporters of reflexology view this stimulation at the ends or periphery of the body as capable of relieving congestion (as congestion is interpreted in traditional Asian systems of care), restoring or rebalancing energy, or acting as a stimulus toward self-healing.

Besides manual movements, reflexologists may sometimes use props such as balls or sticks to stimulate outer body parts. As with other therapies rooted in Asia, the client wears comfortable, loose clothing during a session. Evidence for the effectiveness of reflexology as a stand-alone therapy is not definitive; however, the nontoxic practice may have greater value as an integrative method when used alongside other therapies, especially for the conditions given below.

Reflexology may be useful for stress and anxiety disorders, chronic pain, dementia, diabetes, multiple sclerosis; in eldercare and as caregiver support; and during cancer or palliative care.

MANIPULATIVE METHODS

The most common types of manipulative bodywork include osteopathic manipulation, chiropractic, and Rolfing.

Osteopathy

Four major techniques are used in the whole-person approach to osteopathic diagnosis and treatment: 1) soft tissue manipulation of muscles and connective tissues; 2) osteopathic maneuvers that involve moving or toggling joint surfaces; 3) cranial osteopathy using rhythmic manual compression of the head, neck, and spinal areas; and 4) organ or visceral manipulation using gentle manual pressure directed toward deeper organ tissues.

Osteopathic techniques can also include stimulation of the lymphatic circulation and thrusting or leveraging movements that tend to be rapid yet less forceful or high-speed than chiropractic methods. Techniques such as counterforce or counterstrain are used to treat tender points, aiming to stretch and stimulate tissues to restore mobility and homeostasis (or balance).

Osteopathic manipulative therapy appears useful in acute and chronic lower back pain, back pain associated with pregnancy, other pain and strain conditions, migraine headaches, and carpal tunnel syndrome to potentially delay or prevent surgery.

Osteopathic manipulative techniques may also be useful for irritable bowel syndrome and as part of integrated care for in-hospital pneumonia. The use of these methods in infant colic and pediatrics remains mostly anecdotal or unproven.

Chiropractic

Chiropractic manipulation is often known as an adjustment. These treatments aim to ease tightness or pain and to restore mobility to joints and other musculoskeletal structures through the use of a quick, controlled force to a joint or to the joints in the spine by a chiropractic professional specially trained in these techniques.

Chiropractors use adjustment methods in the belief that the off-centered alignment of the spine causes other imbalances in the body such as alterations in nerve flow that may be the root cause of pain or a variety of other conditions. Once alignment has been restored, the body is then able to heal itself, according to chiropractic beliefs.

Practitioners apply manual pressure after positioning the clothed or gowned client on an examination table. The sudden hand movements can push a joint to its limits of motion, sometimes causing a click or pop that you can hear or feel.

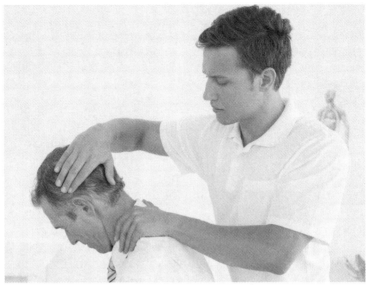

A chiropractor performing an adjustment on a client.

Dozens of chiropractic techniques are in use, many of which are named for the practitioner who developed or popularized them. Some techniques involve the use of special instruments, activators, triangular blocks, or drop tables. Ask what technique your chiropractor intends to use and what you can expect to experience.

People with fragile or weak bones or blood vessels, nerve disorders, bleeding problems, tumors, a risk or history of stroke, dislocations, or fractures can be at higher risk for complications and may not be suited for chiropractic care.

Stroke is a complication that may occur rarely in association with chiropractic manipulation, although mainstream medical practitioners often cite it. In reality, according to older studies reported in the 1980s and 1990s as well as insurance industry reports, the risk of stroke is about one or two in a million manipulations. Higher risks may be seen with neck chiropractic manipulations or perhaps with movements that produce greater twisting motions.

Discuss your treatment options and risk concerns with your doctor and your chiropractor to find the safest, most suitable, and—ideally—more effective option. Multiple chiropractic adjustments, sometimes as many as 30 treatments, may be recommended to you. Consider the need for and the potential expense of such a care plan. You may achieve your maximal benefit in fewer treatments.

Chiropractic care has been shown to be useful for lower back pain and can also be helpful in neck pain. See Chapter 10 for more information about chiropractic care.

Rolfing

Developed in the early to mid-twentieth century, Rolfing, sometimes called the structural integration method, takes its name from its founder, biochemist Ida Rolf. Manual or elbow forces are applied to the body with more pressure than most forms of massage but without the sudden, forceful thrusts associated with chiropractic manipulation. The force is firm and gradual and is applied to the tissue until the target area is felt to give, which is believed to release the tension or adhesions, considered to result in connective tissues that are more supple or elastic.

You may also hear practitioners speak of lengthening tissues, which is interpreted as occurring when the tissues are rendered more pliable or flexible through Rolfing techniques. Many practitioners also introduce clients to biomechanical training of their bodies to improve their alignment against the forces of gravity, to improve posture, and to develop ways of moving or shifting the body that are less stressful.

Evidence for the effectiveness of Rolfing remains preliminary; however, it has been used for anxiety and musculoskeletal disorders, chronic fatigue disorders, to improve balance or gait disturbances, and to foster wellness.

OTHER TECHNIQUES

Alexander Technique

In contrast to many passive bodywork methods, this method relies on guided instruction by the practitioner and the active participation of the client. Trained Alexander providers offer education intended to enhance body awareness so that clients may move, sit, stand, transfer, and otherwise position themselves in ways that minimize or reduce the stresses on the body.

Developed in the late 1800s, Alexander may be taught one-on-one or in groups with no disrobing required. Through activities such as bending, reaching, and other movements, instructors give feedback to help clients achieve better balance and control over their posture and to improve the quality of their movements.

Instructors use their hands and bodies to help guide clients, who are expected to be more active and engaged than in other types of bodywork. This type of nontoxic therapy may be helpful for people with vision problems who can benefit from the instructor's hands-on guidance and supervision, or possibly in certain movement disorders, as in the earlier stages of Parkinson's disease. Studies are underway comparing this technique with acupuncture and usual care for chronic neck pain.

The Alexander technique may also be useful for balance, instability, movement disorders, rehabilitation after injury, stiffness, weakness and fatigue, and chronic neck or back pain.

Feldenkrais Method

Another type of awareness-through-movement method, Feldenkrais aims to retrain the mind-body connection to develop better flexibility and movement coordination.

Also often taught in groups, practitioners use their hands to guide clients in replacing ingrained, less-desirable habits toward more healthful, functional movement patterns, known as functional integration. Although the method has been used for different musculoskeletal conditions as well as for tension, depression, and other ailments, evidence to date about its effectiveness is scant. A study in women with chronic pain reported that despite its benefits, the method's exercises could be difficult for some people to perform or might be considered tough to maintain as part of a regular care regimen.

WHERE TO LEARN MORE

Use these websites to explore and learn more about the different types of bodywork, to locate a therapist, and to find out about your state's licensing or certification requirements.

American Massage Therapy Association: *www.amtamassage.org*

Association of Bodywork & Massage Professionals: *www.massagetherapy.com*

Rolf Institute of Structural Integration: *www.rolf.org*

The Feldenkrais Institute: *www.feldenkraisinstitute.com*

American Society for the Alexander Technique: *http://www.amsatonline.org*

American Chiropractic Association: *www.acatoday.org*

American Osteopathic Association: *www.osteopathic.org*

9

Herbal Products and Dietary Supplements

OVERVIEW

THE PLANT KINGDOM HAS BEEN A SOURCE OF MEDICINAL HEALING FOR PEOPLE around the planet over thousands of years. Even today, an estimated 80% of the world's population use botanicals as medicines. Herbal medicines differ in many ways from conventional Western prescription and nonprescription (over-the-counter) medications. First, being derived from natural plants, herbal products are generally not purified down to a specific chemical that behaves in a known and often predictable way in most people, as occurs with many prescription drugs. Rather, botanicals can often contain different parts of the plant or have a variety of **phytochemicals** that in turn may have very complex, incompletely understood, or unknown ways of behaving in the body. Like prescription products, botanicals and dietary supplements may act differently in different states of health or illness or may behave differently in certain populations.

Second, because botanical products in the U.S. are regulated in an altogether different way from prescription drugs (discussed in depth in Chapter 3), it can be difficult or impossible for consumers to know whether or not their botanical product of choice contains the part of the plant that is believed to contain the active ingredients—and in what proportion, potency, or purity.

Third, whereas modern medicine's drugs are given to target a certain symptom or illness, botanicals are often prescribed by alternative and integrative practitioners in consideration of the individual patient's overall condition, including his or her energetics and constitutional makeup.

Fourth, as with pharmaceutical drugs that can be prepared as pills, capsules, injectables, patches, and in other forms—such as sublingual, or under-the-tongue formulations—herbal medicines have many distinctive forms, too. For example, fresh and dried herbs may also be taken in liquid forms, as in infusions, decoctions, tinctures, and extracts.

Infusions are usually made like a tea—that is, by steeping the flowery or above-ground parts of the plant in a liquid, usually hot water, aiming to dissolve or incorporate the desired ingredients into the liquid. Examples include herbal teas and chamomile.

Decoctions involve boiling parts of the plant—often the woody parts, bark, or roots—to extract its herbal essences.

To help extract the desired plant components, solvents may also be used, such as alcohol or vinegar. The resulting liquid is called a **tincture**, which, being more concentrated, may be more palatable and easier to imbibe than teas or decoctions.

When a certain type of liquid or combination of liquids is used to extract specific plant components, the resulting liquid is called an **extract**. After extractions, these tinctures or extracts can be dried or further processed into pills, capsules, or other forms.

The Supplement Facts Label

Makers of dietary supplements are required to provide consumers with certain information on the Supplement Facts label of their products. This label is usually found on the back of the package and looks something like this example of a krill oil preparation:

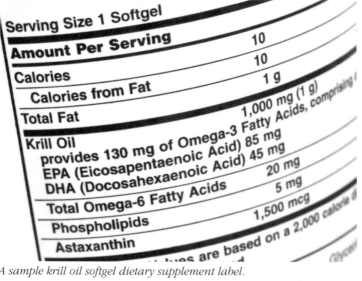

A sample krill oil softgel dietary supplement label.

Source: *www.fda.gov*

Unlike the Nutrition Facts labels for foods, the Supplement Facts label must list ingredients for which no recommended daily intake or daily value (DV) has been established. Moreover, the part of the plant from which the ingredient derives must also be listed on the Supplement Facts label.

The serving size suggested by the manufacturer must also be listed. While the serving size should be the maximum recommended amount you should take at each eating interval, you and your practitioner may decide on a different amount that is safe and appropriate for you.

The label should include the contents of the supplement, the amount of the active ingredients per serving and any other added ingredients such as fillers, flavorings, or preservatives. The disclosure of any key allergens such as gluten is required. Labels for extracts must also identify the solvent used either on the label or on the ingredients list.

The front or more prominent area of a supplement's package offers other information, some of which is designed to sell the product or attract your attention. Despite their appeal, the terms "pharmaceutical grade" and "natural" have no legal definition. Preparations that are manufactured to legitimate, documented, and traceable pharmaceutical grade are generally sold as prescription drugs, not as supplements.

For any label that claims that the product offers some type of nutritional support—for example, "promotes a healthy prostate" or "supports joint health"—the FDA requires all supplement makers to include this disclaimer prominently on the label:

> *These statements have not been evaluated by the Food and Drug Administration. This product is not intended to diagnose, treat, cure, or prevent any disease.*

The Most Popular Supplements

Americans' hunger for dietary supplements continues to grow. According to 2013 data from the *Nutrition Business Journal*, dietary supplements—vitamins, minerals, herbals, amino acids, enzymes, and other products—accounted for $35 billion in consumer spending. What's more, the supplement industry is projected to grow by about 7% a year.

Although supplement fads come and go, certain supplements have dominated in terms of sales and popularity. These have been the 10 best-selling supplements in the U.S. over more than a decade (1997–2012), according to 2012 data from the *Nutrition Business Journal*:

1. Multivitamins
2. Sports nutrition powders and formulas
3. B vitamins
4. Calcium
5. Fish and other animal oils
6. Vitamin C
7. Homeopathic preparations
8. Probiotics
9. Glucosamine/chondroitin
10. Vitamin D

In a survey released by independent, for-profit ConsumerLab in 2015 of 10,000 people who mostly took at least six supplements daily, the top supplements were fish oil and multivitamins, followed by coenzyme Q10, vitamin D, B vitamins, magnesium, calcium, probiotics, and vitamin C.

The results of studies, positive and negative, as well as different types of media exposure have influenced consumer trends in the use of certain supplements (as shown in these two graphs from the 2012 National Health Interview Survey on the facing page).

Next, we'll take a closer look at different types of dietary supplements by category, starting with nutritionals.

Supplement Categories

Most dietary supplements fall into one or more of the following categories.

Nutritionals (including combination or "multi" formulations)

Vitamins
Minerals
Amino acids
Nutritional oils
Prebiotics
Probiotics
Enzymes

Herbals (also known as botanicals; examples: echinacea and ginkgo)

Hormonal products (example: DHEA or dehydroepiandrosterone)

Adaptogens (examples: ginseng and Ashwagandha)

Use of Complementary Health Approaches in the U.S.
National Health Interview Survey (NHIS)

10-YEAR USE TRENDS FOR INDIVIDUAL NON-VITAMIN, NON-MINERAL NATURAL PRODUCTS

PERCENT OF ALL ADULTS REPORTING USE OF THE NATURAL PRODUCT ON THE NHIS

	Milk Thistle	EGCC (Green Tea)	Ginkgo	Ginseng	Echinacea	Glucosamine/ Chondroitin	Melatonin	Probiotics/ Prebiotics	Fish Oil/ Omega-3
2002	NA	NA	4	4.6	7.6	2.8	NA	NA	2.2
2007	0.4	0.7	1.3	1.5	2.2	3.2	0.6	0.4	4.8
2012	0.4	0.6	0.7	0.7	0.9	2.6	1.3	1.6	7.8

NA: Not available.

8-YEAR USE TRENDS* FOR INDIVIDUAL NON-VITAMIN, NON-MINERAL NATURAL PRODUCTS

SALES IN MILLIONS OF DOLLARS FOR NATURAL PRODUCTS

	Milk Thistle	EGCC (Green Tea)	Ginkgo	Ginseng	Echinacea	Glucosamine/ Chondroitin	Melatonin	Probiotics/ Prebiotics	Fish Oil/ Omega-3
2003	66	76	120	95	172	795	62	NA	188
2007	93	139	107	95	126	831	93	366	695
2011	108	157	90	80	117	735	196	760	1145

NA: Not available.

*Nutrition Business Journal, Supplement Business Reports.
Source: National Health Interview Survey, 2012, U.S. Department of Health and Human Services.
Credit: National Center for Complementary and Integrative Health, NIH.

DIETARY SUPPLEMENTS

Açaí

Other names: Acai, Amazonian palm berry.

Used for: Weight loss, anti-aging, antioxidant; immune or digestive enhancement.

Evidence: Anti-cancer, anti-inflammatory, antioxidant activities (in the laboratory). An uncontrolled 2011 pilot study in 10 overweight adults showed improvements in laboratory values related to metabolic syndrome but no significant changes in body size or blood pressure. Larger, definitive studies are scarce.

Safety: Although acai is consumed as a fruit or juice in Latin America, the safety of acai in supplement form remains unknown.

Forms: Tablets, capsules, powders, juices.

Common dose: Varies with preparation; ranges from 50 mg to 2,000 mg per daily serving.

Precautions: Some preparations may be combined with caffeine or stimulant laxatives. Extracts vary in potency with brand-to-brand variations in strength. Some manufacturers have been sued for making false claims about acai's health benefits. Because the acai pulp is used experimentally as a contrast agent, inform your health-care provider if you use acai prior to having an MRI.

Aloe Vera

The gel of this pointy-leaved desert plant has been used for wounds and skin conditions for thousands of years. Today, it is used in a wide range of products, including cosmetics and sunblocks.

Other names: Aloe, lily of the desert.

Used for: Arthritis, skin conditions (topically, applied to the skin for burns, sunburn, psoriasis, herpes, superficial wounds, inflammation) and for laxative effects (when taken by mouth). Aloe was used in traditional healing for parasites, infections, high blood pressure, and diabetes.

Evidence: Best for superficial wounds such as abrasions and burns. Emerging evidence exists for aloe's usefulness in dental hygiene and periodontal health as an anti-plaque, anti-gingivitis agent, as well as for mouth ulcers, cold sores, and lichen planus. Other uses are not well supported. Does not appear to be protective when used to prevent skin damage from radiation therapy.

Safety: Excellent safety when used on the skin for superficial wounds or burns. Oral whole-leaf aloe extract containing latex has been associated with cancer of the bowel in laboratory rodents, but not thus far in humans. Although aloe produces a strong laxative effect when taken orally, aloe can no longer be sold as an over-the-counter laxative because of safety concerns and the need for increasing doses to obtain the desired effect.

Forms: Gel, ointment, and cream (for topical use); tincture (10% aloe vera gel in alcohol); softgels; capsules; juice.

Common dose: 50–200 mg aloe (for constipation).

Precautions: The use of aloe vera dates back to ancient Mesopotamia. Because it can lower blood sugar and blood fats, oral aloe must be used with caution in diabetics and in people taking lipid-lowering medicines. Although short-term use for its laxative properties appears relatively safe, it must be used with caution in people taking diuretics (water pills), medicines that may decrease potassium, or digoxin, or in people with kidney or heart problems—especially due to product variability. Start with small doses of purified preparations, or stick to gel preparations.

Ashwagandha

See Chapter 10 for information about ashwagandha.

Black Cohosh

Black cohosh supplements made from the *Cimicifuga racemosa* plant may contain more than 50 different chemically active substances, and their effects may vary widely depending on the species, preparation, or dose used.

Other names: Rattleweed.

Used for: Relief of menopausal symptoms (hot flashes, vaginal dryness, mood disorders) or related conditions (bone thinning or osteoporosis); premenstrual syndrome (PMS) or menstrual cramps; infertility.

Evidence: Did not appear to work better than placebo for hot flashes in a 2012 Cochrane review, although some studies have shown relief of sweats, especially in women whose symptoms are related to the presence of fibroids (benign tumors of the uterus) and in European studies that used standardized preparations. Possibly effective during short-term use (six months or less) for menopausal mood swings under medical supervision using standardized preparations (from Germany).

Safety: Many international agencies have warned about liver toxicity after reports of serious liver failure. However, many of the products used were adulterated or did not contain black cohosh at all. Product consistency and safety are ongoing concerns.

Forms: Extracts, whole-herb, and root powder forms; the dose required of extracts is usually less than that of other forms.

Common dose: 20 mg (standardized extract) once or twice per day.

Precautions: Potentially serious liver toxicity should still be considered; may cause stomach upset and other general complaints, including sleepiness; not for use in adolescents, pregnant or breast-feeding women, or women with a history of or at high risk for breast cancer. Interactions with sedatives, tranquilizers, and drugs for high blood pressure and cholesterol are possible.

Bromelain

The stem and fruit of the pineapple plant have been used medicinally by many different native cultures throughout the tropical and subtropical regions of the world.

Other names: Pineapple extract, pineapple enzyme, plant protease concentrate.

Used for: Arthritis, inflammation, nasal/sinus congestion, cardiovascular and clotting disorders, muscle aches, digestion, cancer. Also used topically (on the skin) for wounds or burns.

Evidence: Appears helpful for nasal/sinus congestion when used with other conventional medications. Topical bromelain may help the shedding of dead skin resulting from burns, but it is unclear whether bromelain actually helps in burn or wound treatment. Evidence for bromelain's use in osteoarthritis or post-exercise muscle soreness is unsettled.

Safety: Appears relatively safe in humans; allergic reactions may occur. There have been some reports of increased heart rate, digestive problems, and menstrual abnormalities.

Forms: Tablet, capsule, cream, powder.

Common dose: Variable; see label instructions.

Precautions: Bromelain contains a combination of biochemicals that break down proteins (known as proteolytic enzymes) obtained from the stem and juice of pineapples. Bromelain has also been used as a meat tenderizer. Bromelain may increase the absorption of certain antibiotics such as tetracycline and amoxicillin, and perhaps other drugs as well, including blood thinners or tranquilizers.

Butterbur

Leaves of this shrub were used as protective wrapping for butter. Along with the leaves, minus the butter, other parts of the plant have had many uses in folk traditions.

Other names: Petasites, branded names.

Used for: Nasal and seasonal allergies, hay fever and runny nose (rhinitis), allergic reactions (skin), asthma, migraine headaches.

Evidence: Good evidence for its use for nasal and seasonal allergy symptoms such as itchy eyes and rhinitis; established evidence for migraine headache prevention. Butterbur does not appear effective for asthma or skin allergic reactions.

Safety: Well tolerated overall; may cause burping or mild gastrointestinal distress or allergic reactions in people who are allergic to ragweed or other plant and flower allergens.

Forms: Tablets (butterbur extract), extract creams for topical use (on the skin).

Common dose: 75 mg twice daily (for migraine prevention), 50–75 mg twice daily for other uses.

Precautions: Rare cases of hepatitis have been reported with long-term use, which appear to have been caused by the presence of certain chemicals (pyrrolizidine alkaloids—abbreviated PA). Choose supplements that are certified and labeled as PA-free. Be cautious with long-term use, and discuss any persistent headache symptoms with your health-care provider.

Cinnamon

Once a heavily traded and highly cherished spice now treasured in ethnic kitchens throughout the world, the bark of the cinnamon tree has historically been used for a number of ailments.

Other names: Cassia (or Chinese) cinnamon, cinnamon bark, Ceylon cinnamon.

Used for: Traditionally for gastrointestinal disorders, diabetes, colds, energy/appetite stimulation, circulation, and for the *kapha* type in Ayurveda.

Evidence: Cassia cinnamon use may help lower blood sugar; most evidence is inconclusive for other conditions (for example, stomach upset, menstrual problems).

Safety: Appeared safe in a small human trial using up to 6 grams (g) per day for six weeks.

Forms: Capsules (preferred), powders.

Common dose: Varies; the most appropriate dose has not been established. Doses of 1–6 g (equal to about 1–2 teaspoons) have been used to help lower blood sugar.

Precautions: Cinnamon, especially Chinese (cassia) cinnamon, also contains significant amounts of coumarin, the parent compound of the blood thinner warfarin. Use with extreme caution in liver disease or with other medications or herbals that might damage the liver. Taking cinnamon along with other blood sugar–lowering medications may cause potentially dangerous low blood sugar levels or variable blood sugar swings. The supplement form appears preferred over the spice form.

Coenzyme Q10 (CoQ10)

CoQ10 is not considered an **essential nutrient** because it is made by the energy-producing mitochondria—the cellular batteries—of human heart, pancreas, kidney, and liver cells. Although levels of CoQ10 naturally decline with age, it remains overall unclear whether supplementing the diet with CoQ10 can slow or prevent many age-related conditions. Certain foods contain small amounts of CoQ10, including meats, poultry, fish, and some plant-based foods such as soybeans, nuts, and canola oil.

Other names: CoQ10, coenzyme Q, ubiquinone, ubiquinol (the latter are two different forms of the fat-soluble antioxidant).

Used for: Statin-related muscle aches or weakness, heart health, heart failure, high blood pressure, Parkinson's disease (PD); less commonly used for multiple conditions, including headache prevention (migraine), cancer, infertility, HIV, anti-aging, athletic performance, and memory.

Evidence: Good for lowering blood pressure but results are inconsistent regarding heart failure; although earlier studies of early Parkinson's disease showed that high CoQ10 doses (up to 1200–2400 mg per day) may have helped slow progression of the disease, a 2014 multicenter study showed no benefit, despite being well tolerated.

Safety: A natural, vitamin-like chemical made in the mitochondria of human cells, CoQ10 is important in energy production. Although generally very well tolerated, with only rare serious side effects, CoQ10 has the potential for interaction with some blood-thinning medications (warfarin) and may lower blood pressure or glucose.

Forms: Softgels, tablets, capsules, liquids; oil-based or solubilized forms may be better absorbed.

Common dose: 100 mg three times per day for heart failure along with a conventional drug regimen or to prevent migraine; 50–100 mg twice daily for high blood pressure; up to 300 mg daily for statin-related muscle problems or migraine prevention, which may require use for up to three months to achieve preventive effects.

Precautions: Absorption and bioavailability differ among various preparations and individuals. Take dry capsules or tablets with a fatty meal to improve your body's ability to absorb and use CoQ10 efficiently, known as its bioavailability. Instead of taking your dose at one time, spread it out—for example, take it two or three times per day.

Curcumin

See Chapter 10 for information about curcumin and turmeric.

Dehydroepiandrosterone (DHEA)

A powerful steroid hormone, the body converts DHEA to testosterone, estrogen, and other hormones, but to variable degrees in different people. Banned in the mid-1980s, DHEA was back on shelves by a special allowance made in 1994, making it the only over-the-counter steroid permitted to be sold in the U.S.

Other names: DHEA, prasterone, androstenolone.

Used for: Anti-aging, bone and muscle building, menstrual/hormonal problems, weight loss, depression, mental and immune boosting, schizophrenia, slowing of Parkinson's/Alzheimer's diseases, sexual enhancement, overall well-being, lupus, and other disorders.

Evidence: Possible small increase in bone density in women; might offer some benefit in lupus, but its use should be carefully monitored; evidence is inconclusive or conflicting for all other possible indications.

Safety: Possibly safe for short-term, low-dose use, but side effects can include acne, facial hair growth, and voice deepening (in women); high blood pressure; increased heart rate or abnormal heart rhythm; increased aggression; lowering of HDL ("good" cholesterol); mood disorders; menstrual changes; liver damage; blood sugar fluctuations; headache; and insomnia.

Forms: Capsules, tablets, injections, cream.

Common dose: For most indications, 25–50 mg daily; for bone density, 50–100 mg daily.

Precautions: DHEA is a powerful hormone that is naturally produced in humans in the adrenal glands and made into sex hormones in the body. Over-the-counter DHEA is made from wild yam and soy; however, our bodies cannot make DHEA from the yam- and soy-containing foods we eat. As with other hormones, the effects of DHEA can vary widely from one person to another. Use with extreme caution and under the care of a qualified practitioner if you have cancer or diabetes, or if you are taking other hormonal substances (including some types of chemotherapy), insulin, drugs for depression, or other prescription drugs. Also, use with caution with other herbs (for example, ginger, ginkgo, ginseng, and others), licorice, and soy. The use of DHEA is banned by most sporting world agencies and is only available with a prescription in Canada and many other countries. DHEA should not be used by children and pregnant or breast-feeding women.

Echinacea

Although echinacea is an often-used herbal product in the U.S., evidence for its usefulness is surprisingly limited and its use has declined.

Other names: Coneflower, purple or American coneflower; *Echinacea purpurea.*

Used for: Immune support, colds, respiratory infections, flu; also used in traditional healing for wound and skin problems.

Evidence: Equivocal; possible mild effectiveness for common cold severity or duration. One randomized, placebo-controlled study in 755 people showed evidence for cold prevention and symptom relief when echinacea was taken for four months throughout the cold season and during the cold episode using a standardized Swiss-made extract of 2,400–4,000 mg per day in three to five divided doses.

Safety: Occasional mild gastrointestinal upset but overall well tolerated when taken by mouth; can cause serious allergy, asthmatic, or life-threatening anaphylaxis reactions. **Herb-drug interactions** have been reported.

Forms: Tablets, chewable tablets, liquid-filled capsules, tinctures, extracts, powders, tea.

Common dose: Varies according to plant or plant parts used; best taken two to three times per day rather than as one dose during cold season.

Precautions: Reconsider using echinacea if you are allergic to plant members of the daisy family (chrysanthemums, marigolds, and ragweed), if you have asthma or a history of skin reactions (atopy), or if you have a history of an immune disorder or HIV. Echinacea may slow the breakdown of caffeine, possibly causing symptoms such as jitteriness or palpitations. Check for interactions with any prescription drugs you are taking. Preparations may contain different amounts or plant parts of at least three different species, whose individual actions and effectiveness remain unknown. Most studies that have shown some benefit for colds used the above-ground or aerial part of the *Echinacea purpurea* plant. Not recommended for use in young children, pregnant or breast-feeding women, or women who may become pregnant because adequate safety data is lacking.

Fish Oil

The effectiveness of fish oil, the most popular supplement behind vitamins and minerals, with regard to heart health and some other conditions such as arthritis can vary with the dose and the specific condition. Although many recent studies have brought the effectiveness of fish oil into question for heart health, one thing is certain: eating a diet rich in fish, once or twice a week, has been associated with fewer heart events, decreased stroke risk, better health, and lower death rates. Talk to your health-care team about which and how much fish oil might be right for you and how to get the benefits of fish through diet. Good fatty fish sources include salmon, sardines, anchovies, mackerel, bluefish, herring, lake trout, and even canned tuna (the "chunk light" variety may be a better choice with regard to mercury). Overconsumption of certain fish can lead to excess exposure to mercury, a contaminant that is bound to fish flesh but not to the oils. Supplements are generally free from mercury contamination. As with other supplements, look for the USP Verified Mark (read more about this in Chapter 3).

Alpha-linolenic acid, or ALA—the essential omega-3 fatty acid found in plant-based foods such as walnuts, flax, canola oil, and soy—is converted to the two omega-3 fatty acids that have been associated with the majority of fish oil's healthful effects (EPA and DHA, or eicosapentaenoic and docosahexaenoic acids, respectively), but only at a very low rate.

Other names: Omega-3 fatty acids, marine oils.

Used for: Heart and vascular health, arthritis, dry eye, high blood triglycerides, mental functioning/neuroprotection, depression, liver support (nonalcoholic fatty liver disease), bone health (osteoporosis), diabetes, high blood pressure, as add-on therapy in cancer care (preliminary), attention-deficit disorders (example, ADHD).

Evidence: At the correct dose, effective in reducing very high triglyceride levels under a doctor's care; modestly reduces blood pressure; higher doses appear effective in rheumatoid arthritis but less so in osteoarthritis; possibly effective for heart health after a heart attack (to decrease irregular rhythms and sudden death), cardiac atherosclerosis (hardening of the arteries feeding the heart), ADHD, osteoporosis, Raynaud's disease not due to certain collagen diseases, childhood asthma, and for lowering diabetes risk; did not appear effective in a recent study of age-related macular degeneration (AMD).

Safety: Appears overall safe in nonallergic people; some people with depression or bipolar disorder may experience worsening of their symptoms; most common side effects are gastrointestinal, including "fish burps," which can be decreased by keeping capsules or liquids in the refrigerator or freezer, by taking fish oil just before a meal, and by avoiding carbonated drinks.

Forms: Liquids, capsules, softgels, enteric-coated softgels, chewables.

Common dose: 1 g (EPA + DHA) per day for heart health; 2–4 g per day for very high triglycerides (under a doctor's care); variable doses of 1–3 g daily for general health, arthritis, mood disorders, dry eye, and other conditions listed above.

Precautions: Very high doses (generally above 2 g per day) may raise LDL ("bad" cholesterol); the sometimes cited risk of bleeding could be theoretical as people on various fish oil doses did not have significantly increased bleeding in trials that examined blood loss in different types of major surgery; use with blood pressure drugs can lower blood pressure to undesirable levels. Read the label carefully to determine how much EPA and DHA you are getting from a serving and how many capsules constitute a serving. Nearly all of the health benefits of fish oil have been associated with EPA and DHA, not omega-9 and other types of omega fatty acids. Krill oil appears promising but is expensive, and studies on this oil are limited in comparison to fish oil. Vegetarians may consider algal oil as an alternative.

Ginger

Ginger is used as a spice or food accent, notably in Asian, Caribbean, African, and Middle Eastern cuisines. The ginger root may be sliced and steeped to make a tea. Widely used in Ayurveda, traditional Chinese medicine, and many folk traditions, ginger is also a common home remedy for gastrointestinal distress.

Other names: Zingiber officinale.

Used for: Nausea, upset stomach, motion sickness, premenstrual cramps/syndrome, digestion, immune support; as an anti-inflammatory for arthritis and joint pain; for protection against cancer, infection, diabetes, nervous system diseases.

Evidence: Better for nausea associated with pregnancy but not as strong for nausea due to other conditions (cancer chemotherapy, motion sickness, surgery); appears effective for PMS, possibly in conjunction with zinc supplementation; possibly effective for arthritis when taken internally; topical uses do not appear effective; cancer protection and neuroprotection studies are preliminary, without adequate human trials to date.

Safety: Overall safe; may cause a burning sensation in the mouth, bloating, or heartburn.

Forms: Fresh, dried, or roasted root; powder; extract; tea; juice; topical; essential oil.

Common dose: Varies; 170 mg daily (extract) for arthritis; 500 mg twice daily for morning sickness (dried); and up to 500 mg four times daily for other conditions.

Precautions: May irritate the skin, or, when taken internally, may lower blood sugar or possibly increase bleeding risk. Be especially careful about using ginger with anti-clotting medicines and nifedipine (a heart drug). Pregnant women with bleeding problems or a history of miscarriages should not take ginger.

Ginkgo

At more than 200 million years old, the *Ginkgo biloba* species is one of the world's oldest living trees and is considered sacred in China. Traditionally, ginkgo the herb has been used for breathing and circulation ailments and is now used for many conditions, despite an overall absence of evidence. Ginkgo has antioxidant, free radical scavenging, and metabolic actions on cell membranes; it also helps with energy production and other activities. Ginkgo is mostly regulated as a prescription herbal medicine in Europe.

Other names: Ginkgo biloba, maidenhair tree.

Used for: Cardiovascular and immune support, intestinal disorders, slowing or preventing Alzheimer's, mental focus or clarity, memory, relief of painful walking due to circulation problems of the legs (intermittent claudication), support during cancer therapy, tinnitus, depression, eye disorders.

Evidence: Nearly all of the reliable studies have shown no positive effects on Alzheimer's prevention or slowing, dementia, and memory or mental functioning. May possibly help some types of dizziness (vertigo due to inner-ear disturbances); does not appear effective for tinnitus and most other disorders.

Safety: Overall well tolerated; the many side effects reported include headaches, dizziness, nausea, gastrointestinal upset, bleeding, and skin allergy—including severe allergic reactions. May interact with anti-clotting medicines (warfarin, aspirin, and others) and anti-diabetic, anti-hypertensive, anti-depressant, or anti-seizure drugs.

Forms: Tablets, capsules, teas

Common dose: Adults can take 120 mg daily of a standardized extract in two or three divided doses.

Precautions: Because of platelet-inhibiting activity, ginkgo may potentially increase bleeding risk and is one of the most common supplements stopped before surgery. Ginkgo is usually not advised for people who have had a stroke or who are at risk for stroke or bleeding problems, although the risk of bleeding may be theoretical. Avoid ginkgo if you take thiazides, a water pill for blood pressure. Chewing or eating raw or roasted seeds may lead to seizures or death. The risk for cancer with long-term use in humans remains unknown, but some cancers have developed in animals fed much higher doses than are usually ingested by people. A significant number of off-the-shelf products tested did not contain the stated amount of ginkgo marker compounds or were spiked with added imitation compounds or fillers. Products with *Ginkgo biloba* leaf extract may be more like the products used in studies, although there is no assurance of batch-to-batch reliability.

Ginseng

A popular herb worldwide, ginseng has a 2,000-year-long history in traditional and folk medicine, notably in traditional Chinese, Korean, and other Asian practices. Most studies of its health benefits have focused on the Asian and American varieties. Siberian ginseng, or *Eleutherococcus senticosus*, is a different plant altogether. Nearly 50 different ginsenosides have been identified in ginseng, which are the major active phytochemicals, although many others with activity in humans exist. Plants contain variable amounts of ginseng, often depending on the plant's age, which part of the plant was harvested, and how the herb is processed.

An **adaptogen**, ginseng is often used as a tonic to boost well-being, energy, resistance to disease, and vitality. Its many uses as a preventive and in many conditions reflect the diverse properties associated with its complex—and highly variable—biochemical composition. Some products may contain little or none of the active ingredients. Ginseng's range of active phytochemicals makes it an attractive herb for further study, especially with improvements to product quality and consistency. Expect more news about ginseng in the future.

Other names: *Panax ginseng* (Asian), *Panax quinquefolius* (American).

Used for: Overall health, anti-aging, immune support, blood sugar (lowering), mental and physical performance, nervous system function, Alzheimer's, lung function, blood pressure control, circulation, sexual function, menopausal symptoms, depression, anxiety, fatigue or chronic fatigue, anti-cancer, and multiple other uses.

Evidence: Possibly effective for mental function and Alzheimer's, lung function (including cystic fibrosis), sexual function, high blood pressure, menopausal symptoms, depression, and to aid in blood glucose control.

Safety: Short-term use appears safe overall, although allergy and herb or drug interactions can occur. Side effects include headaches and gastrointestinal and sleep disturbances. Know that some types of ginseng or ginseng products can unpredictably lower blood sugar, and others may raise it.

Forms: Tablet, capsule, tea, fresh (root slices), extract, powder, tincture, cream, juice, ethnic foods.

Common dose: Varies according to potency and preparation; 100 mg of standardized extract or 1–2 g of root powder.

Precautions: Use caution with other herbs or drugs that may lower blood pressure or blood sugar. As with many herbs with biologic activity, reconsider with your health-care team or avoid using ginseng at all if you are on multiple medications, antidepressants, or antiretrovirals (for HIV), or if you are using powerful anti-clotting drugs such as warfarin.

Glucosamine/Chondroitin

Glucosamine and chondroitin are naturally present in cartilage, the cushioning tissues at the ends of bony moving parts at joints. These supplements are usually taken together and may require a minimum of two to four months of continuous use before effects are noted (if any). The crystalline form of glucosamine sulfate may be the preferred formulation for arthritis over the N-acetyl glucosamine form.

Other names: Chitosamine.

Used for: Osteoarthritis, particularly of the knee and hip.

Evidence: Conflicting, but mostly negative, for halting progression of arthritis. Evidence for improvements in joint pain and mobility is weak, although possible small effects have been shown in some studies. Contrary studies have shown no significant effects, even when standardized doses and formulations were used.

Safety: Appears relatively safe, except for those with a shellfish allergy (both are made from natural cartilage sources); some gastrointestinal side effects have been reported.

Forms: Combination preparations available as capsules, liquids, powders, tablets.

Common dose: Glucosamine 500 mg with chondroitin 400 mg three times daily; may require two to four months of use before producing any effects.

Precautions: Use with caution and under a health-care practitioner's care with anti-clotting medications (warfarin) because of the potential for interaction. Negative potential effects of glucosamine on blood sugar metabolism and in diabetics appear unlikely to occur at usual doses; however, consult your health-care provider.

Magnesium

An essential mineral, magnesium is present in many foods (green leafy vegetables, nuts, beans, legumes, milk, yogurt, soy milk, avocados, some fish, and fortified cereals, among others) as well as in multivitamins and some combination calcium supplements. Although Americans can get enough magnesium from a well-balanced diet, many people may lose magnesium because of laxative use, gastrointestinal or absorption problems, medications (especially proton-pump inhibitors for excess stomach acid), diabetes, advancing age, or excess alcohol consumption. Although healthy kidneys will rid the body of excess magnesium consumed in food, be aware that too much supplemental magnesium may be toxic or cause health problems.

Other names: Magnesium oxide, citrate, gluconate, chloride, malate, lactate, aspartate, and other forms.

Used for: Blood pressure lowering (small effect) and cardiovascular health, diabetes and metabolic syndrome, migraine headache prevention, osteoporosis/bone health, restoring adequate levels in people with alcohol use disorders.

Evidence: Good for migraines; essential for bone health in adequate amounts; promising for pre-diabetes and diabetes, heart health, and possibly stroke prevention, along with other measures.

Safety: Diarrhea may occur with supplements (another form may be better tolerated); do not exceed 100% of the daily value in supplement form unless under a doctor's care (for example, for migraine prevention or if you are deficient due to illness, alcohol use, or medication).

Forms: Tablets, caplets, capsules, powders, softgels, enteric coated, liquids.

Common dose: Varies according to the amount of elemental magnesium in each form; the total recommended daily intake for adults is 320 mg (women) and 420 mg (men).

Precautions: Magnesium can interact or have unwanted effects with certain antibiotics (quinolones, tetracycline), osteoporosis drugs (bisphosphonates), proton-pump inhibitors, and diuretics. Use with caution if you have kidney or heart disease or are on medications for those conditions. Blood tests alone may not be enough to diagnose magnesium deficiency and should be interpreted along with a careful medication, nutritional, substance use, and health history.

Melatonin

This natural hormone plays a role in sleep and has been shown to be useful for jet lag and certain types of sleep problems, such as sleep disorders in shift workers. There isn't enough safety information on the long-term use of melatonin in adults and children. Moreover, the safe and effective uses of melatonin in children overall, which are unregulated uses of the product throughout the world, have not been adequately studied or described.

Other names: Pineal hormone.

Used for: Mostly for sleep disorders and jet lag; less commonly used as an add-on therapy in cancer care; also used in tinnitus, Alzheimer's, and ALS (amyotrophic lateral sclerosis, or Lou Gehrig's disease).

Evidence: Appears effective for jet lag, for trouble falling asleep in younger populations (young adults, possibly children), and for sleep-wake disorders associated with underlying nervous system disease or disabilities; possibly effective for general insomnia, withdrawal from benzodiazepine tranquilizers, anxiety before surgical procedures, and cancer care; does not appear effective for depression.

Safety: Appears safe for short-term use; side effects can include headache, dizziness, nausea, or feeling drowsy or irritable.

Forms: Pills, lozenges, sublingual (under the tongue), liquid, timed-release and buccal (applied inside the cheek) formulations.

Common dose: 0.5–5 mg at bedtime for sleep; for jet lag, 0.5–3 mg on the arrival day to a destination (at least one time zone away; best for eastward travel up to four time zones away) and continued for up to five days; higher doses up to 5 mg are sometimes used.

Precautions: Available only by prescription in many countries including Australia, melatonin may not be safe in pregnant women, infants, or children; the use of melatonin in people with high blood pressure, diabetes, seizures, bleeding disorders, or depression or in transplant recipients may trigger symptoms related to those respective conditions; many prescription drugs and dietary supplements may interact with melatonin, so use with caution and consult with your healthcare team. Begin with lower doses for sleep. Avoid driving or doing potentially hazardous work or activities for about five hours after taking melatonin.

Milk Thistle

Milk thistle extracted from the seeds of *Silybum marianum*, a member of the daisy family, has been used for liver ailments for over a thousand years. Plant extracts contain many different active compounds, including quercetin, which vary in their actions and targets. Milk thistle's protective effects on the heart, liver, and brain may be due to its ability to prime, or precondition, these tissues to withstand the effects of an insult such as ischemia, or an interruption in blood or nutrient flow, that occurs once the injury has been halted and flow has been restored—at least in animal or lab studies.

Other names: Silymarin, St. Mary's thistle.

Used for: Liver protection, non-alcoholic fatty liver disease (NAFLD), hepatitis C, alcoholic hepatitis, cancer prevention (prostate, skin), diabetes, antioxidant and anti-inflammatory effects.

Evidence: Promising for liver protection and for physical functioning in hepatitis C, although unproven or equivocal with respect to benefit in hepatitis C by laboratory or viral measurements; possibly helpful in diabetes and cancer prevention.

Safety: Overall well tolerated; gastrointestinal disturbances can include loose stools and diarrhea; may trigger allergic reactions, especially in people allergic to ragweed, daisies, and other related plants.

Forms: Capsules, tablets, soft gels, liquids, dry seed powder.

Common dose: 200 mg three times daily of a standardized extract; 280–560 mg every eight hours (NAFLD, alcoholic cirrhosis, hepatitis C).

Precautions: Many independently tested milk thistle products had either low concentrations of extract or were not standardized to higher levels (70–80%) of silymarin, the active ingredient. Because it may lower blood sugar, milk thistle should be used cautiously in diabetics or by people who take other medicines or supplements that can lower blood sugar.

Oils

Tea Tree Oil

Australian aboriginal tribes have long used tea tree oil for a variety of skin conditions.

Other names: Tea tree essential oil, Australian tea tree oil, Melaleuca oil.

Used for: As a folk remedy for dandruff, acne, athlete's foot, nail fungus, superficial skin wounds, lice, other skin or mouth lesions (thrush).

Evidence: May be effective or have less side effects than conventional treatments for acne; early studies suggest it may be useful when used alongside conventional therapy for difficult-to-treat skin infections such as MRSA (methicillin-resistant *Staphylococcus aureus*); some positive results for its use in dandruff and fungal infections of the skin (athlete's foot) and nails.

Safety: Skin use may be irritating or cause allergic reactions, but it is overall considered safe for use in adults.

Forms: Topical oil and gel.

Common dose: Applied to skin.

Precautions: Tea tree oil should not be swallowed by mouth, which has led to coma and other serious complications akin to poisoning.

Other Essential Oils

In aromatherapy, the oily and often scent-laden essence of flowers and plants, known as essential oils, are used to enhance well-being— be it spiritual, emotional, or physical. By inhaling the aromas given off by essential oils as they diffuse into the air, the volatile aroma molecules travel up the nose and cause our nervous system's relay system to fire, engaging sensitive areas such as the limbic system, the brain's seat of emotion and pleasure. Aromatherapy is also used in massage or by itself to help relieve stress and anxiety. Essential oils are also applied to the skin or ambient surfaces such as bedding or pillows to help usher in drowsiness and deeper, more restful sleep.

Other names: Lavender, peppermint, ylang ylang, tea tree, rosemary, Patchouli, grapefruit seed extract, geranium, orange, lemongrass, cinnamon, sandalwood, kunzea, sage, oregano, neroli, ginger, and other oils or oil blends.

Used for: General anxiety or tension related to cancer care, stress, and surgery; pain, muscle relaxation, nausea, and vomiting after surgery; disinfection; sleep disorders.

Evidence: Despite widespread beliefs regarding the calming effects of essential oils, the evidence remains patchy at best. Lavender and orange oil may be effective for anxiety, pain, and relaxation; blends of essential oils have been shown to be calming in patients about to receive heart stents. Peppermint, spearmint, and oil combinations appear to relieve nausea and gastrointestinal upset, but evidence is inconsistent.

Safety: Allergic reactions may occur.

Forms: Oils for topical or ambient use.

Common dose: Applied or massaged to skin; drops may be sprayed on bedding for sleep disorders or general relaxation.

Precautions: Do not consume oils internally; sensitization, rash, or more severe allergies may occur (notably reported with the more commonly used oils—that is, lavender, ylang ylang, peppermint, and tea tree oil; see the separate entry regarding tea tree oil).

Probiotics

Interest in and the use of probiotics have soared, both in the U.S. and globally. Unlike other dietary supplements, probiotics are live microorganisms. When they are consumed in sufficient numbers, probiotics are believed to attach themselves to or to inhabit a part of the body, which in humans is the gastrointestinal tract—particularly the colon—for a health benefit.

Probiotics must be distinguished from **prebiotics**, which are nutrients, foods, or food ingredients that are not digested and are beneficial to the survival of probiotic organisms. Products that contain prebiotics along with probiotics are called **synbiotics**.

Considered "friendly bugs," probiotics are also available in foods—typically yogurts with live active cultures, kefir, and other types of milk products that are fermented such as acidophilus milks, buttermilk, and sour cream. Soy-based sources of probiotics include soy yogurts, tempeh, and miso. The Korean condiment kimchi and sauerkraut, as well as many functional foods and beverages, may also contain probiotics.

The most common probiotics on supplement shelves are *Bifidobacteria*, *Lactobacillus*, and *Saccharomyces boulardii*. *Bifidobacteria* and *lactobacilli* are typical inhabitants of the gut, so-called normal flora, whereas *Saccharomyces* is a yeast that does not cause disease in healthy people, an example being brewer's yeast. Many subtypes of these various groups exist. Just how many of each kind of microbe are needed for maximum benefits, in what combination, and for how long they should be taken are unclear. In nonprescription dietary supplement form, the amounts and combinations are not standardized, which makes determining the specific effectiveness of each microbe and their amounts, whether alone or in combination, unchartered territory for your specific condition or health aim.

Probiotics are consumed for a variety of conditions as well as for overall health. The strongest evidence for their usefulness mostly relates to diarrhea—both the sudden, acute type and that associated with taking antibiotics. Because antibiotics can wipe out both abnormal and normal microbes or flora in the gut, probiotics are believed to help restore the balance of beneficial bacteria to the gut.

There is good evidence that taking probiotics can shorten the duration of diarrhea. It also appears that probiotics may decrease the frequency of bowel movements in a person with diarrhea. What is still unclear is how much and what kind of probiotics work best in different groups of people, as well as their safety in special groups such as children, older adults, and people with chronic health conditions or faulty immune systems due to disease or drugs.

Good evidence also supports the use of a prescription probiotic formulation that contains a mixture and standardized amount of many different bacteria for ulcerative colitis and irritable bowel disorders.

Evidence also supports the use of probiotics in certain forms of inflammatory bowel disease. The strongest evidence exists for ulcerative colitis with conflicting and as-yet-undetermined effectiveness for Crohn's disease.

Probiotics are also available in suppository and cream forms. The cream form is sometimes used in infants for a benign skin condition known as atopic eczema. Probiotics in any form should not be used in premature infants without close medical supervision. Infants with immature immune systems may not be able to handle live organisms, whether considered friendly in adults or not. Nonetheless, there is some evidence that probiotics, when used by the health-care team as part of hospital care, may reduce the risk of a dangerous type of intestinal condition called necrotizing enterocolitis that affects premature babies.

In adults, some evidence exists for the use of probiotics in lessening the side effects associated with treatments for the stomach bacteria known as *Helicobacter pylori* that have been linked to the development of ulcers. Some encouraging results have been shown for the use of probiotics for dental health, although evidence for cavity prevention and periodontal disease is inconclusive to date.

Other potential uses for probiotics include immune support, cholesterol and weight management, and possibly uncomplicated respiratory infections or colds. However, proof and safety issues surrounding such uses have not yet been established.

Other names: *Lactobacillus, Bifidobacterium, Saccharomyces, Bacillus*, others.

Used for: Diarrhea, ulcerative colitis/inflammatory bowel disease (IBD), dental health, immune support, lactose intolerance, uncomplicated respiratory infections, overall health.

Evidence: Best for diarrhea, irritable bowel syndrome, and the ulcerative colitis form of IBD.

Safety: Overall safe and well tolerated in generally healthy and non-allergic people with intact immune systems; may cause mild gastrointestinal distress or gas.

Forms: Capsules, tablets, powders, liquids, creams, suppositories, foods.

Common dose: Varies.

Precautions: Should be used under medical supervision in infants, chronically ill children or adults, the elderly, immune-compromised individuals (including HIV/AIDS and cancer patients), and perhaps others. Formulations, potency, and viability of the organisms vary widely; consult an unbiased health-care practitioner or pharmacist for guidance. Store probiotics away from heat and light, and use them within the expiration date. Read the label for any potential allergens, especially if you are allergic to milk or soy. Do not take probiotics containing *Saccharomyces* (notably *Saccharomyces cerevisiae*) if you are taking antifungals, antidepressants, or other medications classified as MAO inhibitors. If you are also taking antibiotics, it is generally recommended to space out your probiotics and antibiotics doses by at least two hours.

Resveratrol

Found in small amounts in certain foods and beverages, notably grapes, wine (red more so than white), berries, dark chocolate, and peanuts, resveratrol has captured the imagination of the wellness and anti-aging communities. Many of the potential benefits of resveratrol have yet to be proven in humans. A 2014 study of nearly 800 elderly Italians living in the Chianti region found that different levels of resveratrol (as measured in the urine) obtained through diet alone did not correlate with blood markers of inflammation, cardiovascular disease, cancer, or the overall death rate over nine years of follow-up. Because this popular polyphenol shows a dramatic range of potential health-promoting effects in animal, cell culture, and test tube studies, the results of more studies can be expected.

Other names: May be extracted from the Japanese knotweed plant, *Polygonum cuspidatum*, or the seeds or skins of grapes.

Used for: Overall health, longevity; protection from diabetes; prevention of degenerative nervous system diseases (Alzheimer's), heart disease, or stroke; anti-aging and anti-cancer activity; weight management.

Evidence: Very limited; most studies have been done in the lab or in animals. Studies in humans have been in small groups and/or short term with conflicting results.

Safety: Appears safe for short-term use but data is incomplete; a study in patients with myeloma, a form of blood cancer, had to be stopped because the experimental resveratrol group developed a type of kidney damage associated with that disease.

Forms: Capsule, softgels, liquids, or as a red wine or grapeseed extract.

Common dose: Varies, 50–350 mg per day in two divided doses with a meal.

Precautions: Despite its wide-ranging promise in the laboratory and certain animal models, human studies have not provided adequate proof of supplemental resveratrol's benefits as claimed. Long-term safety studies are also lacking. Evidence of life extension is largely limited to lower-life forms (yeast and roundworms). If you are a resveratrol-believer, a diet containing blueberries and other resveratrol-rich foods or beverages may be a wiser choice.

St. John's Wort

Depression is a serious condition, especially in its more profound form, known as major depression. Self-care without input and continued interaction with a qualified health professional or team is considered unwise in major depression. The evidence for the usefulness of St. John's wort appears stronger with milder forms of depression. However, because St. John's wort can interact with numerous and so many different types of prescription drugs, it is especially important to discuss the use or considered use of this supplement with your health-care provider. In Germany, where herbal remedies are commonly used but are generally standardized and subject to regulation, St. John's wort is typically dispensed by prescription.

Other names: Hypericum, *Hypericum perforatum.*

Used for: Depression, anxiety, sleep disorders, hot flashes.

Evidence: Appears more effective for mild or moderate forms of depression; does not appear better than a placebo for major depression.

Safety: Multiple drug interactions and cautions apply; see precautions below.

Forms: Tablets, capsules, extracts, teas, topical preparations.

Common dose: 300–1200 mg per day

Precautions: St. John's wort has many known interactions with prescription drugs and probably even more interactions that remain to be discovered. The list of drugs that may interact with St. John's wort includes an array of antidepressants; cough medicines containing dextromethorphan; birth control pills; transplant rejection and immune suppression drugs (cyclosporine, others); statins; anti-retroviral drugs for HIV; digoxin and other drugs for heart disease; muscle relaxants; anti-ulcer and anti-diarrheal drugs; anti-cancer drugs (irinotecan, others); anti-seizure, anti-anxiety, anti-migraine, anti-fungal, and anti-clotting medications. Other known side effects include an increased sensitivity to sunlight, dry mouth, dizziness, constipation, and gastrointestinal upset. A possible association with an increased risk of cataracts has also been reported and remains to be clarified.

Turmeric

See Chapter 10 for information about turmeric and curcumin.

Vitamins

Although taking a multivitamin may seem like a no-brainer that can only help and not harm, the benefits are not as obvious as they may seem. First, most studies that have tried to sort out whether people who take multivitamins are better off than people who do not have not shown a definite benefit to taking them. The absence of a clear-cut benefit was apparent whether the researchers measured the death rate; the incidence of cancer, heart attacks, or stroke; and other outcomes. In fact, a few studies have shown a link between taking vitamin supplements such as vitamin E or vitamin A and an increased risk for prostate or lung cancer, respectively.

Do You Need a Multivitamin?

Like many studies in nutrition and other health concerns, vitamin studies have largely been observational—that is, studies that looked at populations over time to observe the effects of taking or not taking a vitamin or therapy. Observational studies do not prove cause and effect; rather, they report associations unlike certain types of clinical trials that are designed to measure cause and effect.

Observational results may be hard to interpret because the people being studied may make up a skewed subgroup of the population— for example, people who are better educated or who generally have healthier habits, or people who may have been taking different vitamin formulas or may have taken the supplements irregularly.

In contrast, more robust scientific studies or trials tend to look at study participants known as subjects who meet certain criteria so that the slate for the study is as clean as possible. For example, a quality study on a natural product or a new prescription drug would not be designed to lump the results obtained from people who were generally healthy with those from people who were chronically ill into one group.

Also, clinical trials that attempt to decipher whether an effect is present and to what degree with respect to a certain treatment will typically begin with a very specific therapy that is begun in a controlled and organized way in one group. In addition, such studies are designed to compare the results with those obtained from a group that does not receive the therapy to a group that receives a dummy therapy, called the **placebo** control group. Because of these and other problems in the design, execution, and statistical or mathematic interpretation of many observational studies, it can be difficult to translate their results into recommendations that apply to the general public.

Despite such hurdles, a few recommendations have emerged that appear solid, based on the current state of nutritional science. Keep these tips in mind when considering, buying, and taking multivitamins:

- **Endeavor to get your vitamins from food.** Make foods your medicine by choosing foods that are dense in nutrients (and, preferably, not dense in energy—measured as calories), and mix them up regularly to jazz your palate and to provide your body with the range of nutrients it needs.
- **Take your multivitamin with a meal.** Vitamins are contained within foods in their natural state, from which they can be absorbed. Allow your body to extract all their nutrient goodness by taking multivitamins with your meal. Better still, break your multivitamin in half and take each half with a different meal to allow greater absorption and a better-spaced nutrient intake.
- **Get 100% of the daily value of these, but not all, micronutrients.** Even with vitamins, more of a good thing is not necessarily better. While your multi should contain 100% of the daily value (DV) for the B vitamins B1 (thiamin), B2 (riboflavin), B3 (niacin), B12, and folate (in supplement form as folic acid), remember that many foods are enriched with these B vitamins, too. If you are also taking a separate B vitamin supplement, you may be boosting your intake beyond what you need. Too much folic acid may be associated with an increased cancer risk, so be mindful of your Bs. As for minerals, your multi should also provide 100% of your DV needs for chromium, copper, iodine, selenium, and zinc.

- **Avoid high doses of Vitamin A.** Combined doses of Vitamin A from foods and supplements above 6,000 IU (International Units) may place you at greater risk for fracture, particularly when it comes to hip breaks if you are postmenopausal. Because high doses may increase their risk of lung cancer, smokers should also avoid high doses of supplemental beta-carotene, the Vitamin A precursor form found in fruits, vegetables, and supplements, which the body converts to Vitamin A. Food sources of Vitamin A do not appear to carry these added health risks.

- **Know on which side of the iron curtain you fall.** Iron is needed for growth, and many women need the iron boost during the menopausal years. However, most men and postmenopausal women probably do not need supplemental iron, which might even be harmful for heart health and other organ systems. Discuss your iron status with your health-care provider to determine if you're better off skipping iron.

- **Brand or generic multivitamins?** Many generic multis are dependable brands in and of themselves, offering good absorption and a cheaper price tag than name brands. Consult a reliable pharmacist to find the best source for you. Just because a brand may be loaded with megadoses or tricked out with extra herbs, enzymes, or other ingredients may not necessarily mean that you need them or that they will benefit your health.

Genetically Customized Formulas

As more manufacturers hop on the genetics bandwagon, it's not surprising to find that supplements now tout formulations that claim or suggest that they can make up for deficiencies or faults that may lurk in your genes. Claims that have gone too far, including from companies that also required a DNA test from a cheek swab specimen for an extra fee, have tangled with the Federal Trade Commission (FTC) about some of their unscrupulous marketing techniques and misinformation.

Consumers should know that their chances of a finding a genetic match for their highly individual genetic makeup from an over-the-counter product are about as likely as being bitten by a shark after getting hit by lightning during an earthquake. Instead of this genetic roulette, find a qualified practitioner who can competently evaluate your significant individual genetic risks that you can do something about. Together, you can evaluate what modifications might be worth pursuing, including lifestyle factors, which are far more likely to steer you toward better health.

Who Really Needs a Multivitamin or Mineral Supplement?

Certain individuals could benefit from boosting their nutrient intake beyond what's available from foods. If you count yourself as belonging to one of the following groups, discuss any special nutrient needs you may have with your health-care team to determine your best path to health.

- **Vegetarians and vegans**, who may not get enough Vitamin B12 (only available from animal products), along with the minerals calcium, iron, and zinc.
- **Persons over age 60**, whose diets may not be adequately fresh, diverse, or balanced, or who may be chronically ill, on multiple medications, or have diseases that limit their body's ability to get B vitamins and magnesium—found in leafy greens, whole grains, legumes, nuts, and beans.
- **Darker-skinned individuals, heavy sunscreen users, and cold-climate inhabitants**, who may not make enough Vitamin D because of limited exposure to sunlight.
- **People who take multiple medications**, many of which may cause deficiencies in certain vitamins or minerals—from common antibiotics to specialized drugs for gastrointestinal complaints and heart disease.
- **Pregnant and breast-feeding women**, who have greater nutritional requirements for iron, folic acid supplementation, and omega-3 fatty acids, among others.
- **Smokers and people who drink more than two to three drinks per day**, who may not be eating a balanced diet, or in whom vitamin deficiencies are known to occur, as in thiamin (B1) and magnesium deficiencies in heavy drinkers.
- **People on weight-loss, fad, or other special diets** who may not be eating a sufficiently balanced or diverse diet that contains enough essential nutrients, or people on diets that popularize foods or food-like substances, from tropical fats to artificial sweeteners, whose nutritional value could be questioned.

DRUG-SUPPLEMENT INTERACTIONS

As you've already seen, supplements contain a variety of ingredients that have a range of activities in the body. People do, after all, take them because they expect them to have an effect or many effects. Although our understanding of these effects is incomplete, it continues to grow and to be refined.

Reasons for our incomplete knowledge about dietary supplement ingredients include the fact that they are used by people of many different races and conditions who are often taking other drugs or supplements. Finding out how a supplement can be expected to behave in you particularly or in a group of individuals who share a common underpinning such as age group, sex, state of health, or ethnic background, or those who are on a common medicine, is exceedingly difficult. Plus, when the fact that off-the-shelf products such as supplements vary widely in potency and contents is factored in, practically all bets are off in terms of making accurate predictions.

So how should a well-informed health consumer proceed?

- To be safe, do your research about possible drug-herb, herb-herb, and herb-food interactions.
- Use the many drug-herb interaction checkers available online.
- Consider consulting with a pharmacist if your medication and supplement regimen is lengthy or complicated.
- Discuss your findings or concerns with your health-care team.
- Always use extra care if you are taking multiple medications or if you are at risk for serious complications because of your age, overall condition, or other factors.

Fortunately, because health-care professionals, patients, and health-care consumers are able to report side effects or problems with supplements—whether to their health-care team or to the FDA's Medwatch program (by phone, fax, or online)—scientists are learning more about potential side effects, dangers, and interactions with foods, drugs, or other herb or supplement products.

People take supplements because they expect an effect or result. Understand that the state of our knowledge and the unpredictability of the products sold in this country may not always work to your benefit or lead to an improved health status. Seek out reliable information and keep the lines of communication open with your health-care team. Regarding supplements, as with other health decisions, determine first whether your health priorities, nutrition, and lifestyle choices are maximally aligned toward wholesome ways of supporting your well-being. If they are not, a few simple modifications could boost your health quotient well beyond that hoped for from fistfuls of supplements.

WHERE TO LEARN MORE

Office of Dietary Supplements, National Institutes of Health: *www.ods.od.nih.gov*

Herbs at a Glance (the National Center for Complementary and Integrative Health): *www.nccih.nih.gov/health/herbsataglance.htm*

Herb and supplement information from the National Institutes of Health and the Natural Medicines Comprehensive Database: *www.nlm.nih.gov/medlineplus/druginfo/herb_All.html*

Example of an online free drug and drug-herb interaction checker: *www.webmd.com/interaction-checker/*

A safety information and side effects reporting program of the U.S. Food and Drug Administration, telephone 1-888-INFO-FDA (1-888-463-6332): *http://www.fda.gov/Safety/MedWatch/*

Ingredient and supplement monographs and natural product information in the Licensed Natural Health Products Database from Health Canada: *www.hc-sc.gc.ca*

Fee- or Subscription-based Information:

Consumer Lab (includes specific brand information and regular updates): *www.consumerlab.com*

Consumer version of the Natural Medicines Comprehensive Database: *http://naturaldatabaseconsumer.therapeuticresearch.com/*

Evidence-graded information on natural products and integrative therapies: *https://naturalmedicines.therapeuticresearch.com/*

10

Integrated Approaches: From Ancient to Modern

MANY DIFFERENT TYPES OF HEALING SYSTEMS HAVE ARISEN AND EVOLVED independently of the type of care and philosophies upon which modern, technology-driven medicine are based.

As described in Chapter 6, traditional Chinese medicine began thousands of years ago, spawning variations throughout different parts of Asia. Among other whole systems of care that have developed are ancient healing arts such as Ayurveda. Other, more recent comprehensive approaches to health have only been fleshed out in the last century or two. This chapter begins with perhaps the oldest of these traditional healing arts, Ayurveda.

AYURVEDA

The name of this traditional healing system, often translated as "the science of life," comes from the ancient Sanskrit words *ayur*, meaning life, and *veda*, or knowledge. Originally passed down as an oral tradition, Ayurveda was recorded as far back as 1500 B.C.E in sacred Hindu texts known as The Vedas.

Harmony is essential to health in Ayurvedic beliefs, in which all living things along with earthly objects and the universe itself are made up of five basic elements—air, earth, fire, water, and space— sometimes called ether or vacuum.

From an Ayurvedic perspective, life is viewed holistically in an integrated context that embodies many levels of being. The universal interconnectedness of Ayurveda takes into account not just the physical but also the mental, spiritual, social, familial, and other facets of human existence, including kind and compassionate behaviors.

These interconnected parts of our existence are also linked to our physical constitution known as *prakriti*, which reflects the balance or imbalance of the three life forces, or *doshas*. These doshas are *pitta* (fire), *kapha* (earth and water), and *vata* (air and space). A healthy state is when an individual's unique combination of doshas is in harmony, supported by a clear and peaceful mind along with body tissues that function harmoniously.

Because an individual's dosha reflects a multifaceted blueprint of that person's emotional, physical, and mental state, the restorative belief in lifestyle changes to address prevention, imbalances, and illness is central to Ayurvedic beliefs. Nourishment and eating habits are also important in Ayurveda, which considers food as medicine.

Know Your Doshas

In Ayurveda, each of us has a unique combination or dominance of doshas. Doshas change and morph, intensifying and contracting along with our life experiences, development, events, diet, and activities. This table offers a simple starting point for understanding your individual blend of life forces according to Ayurvedic teachings.

Dosha	Manifests	Associations
Vata (air, space)	Slender build	Constipation
		Dry or rough skin
		Restlessness
		Dislikes cold weather
		Creativity
When balanced/imbalanced		Enthusiasm/anxiety
Pitta (fire)	Medium or muscular build	Warm-bodied
		Fair skin
		Inflammation
		Dislikes warm weather
		Sharp mind
When balanced/imbalanced		Contentment/jealousy
Kapha (earth, water)	Larger build	Indigestion or congestion
		Moist or oily skin
		Deliberate or pensive
		Dislikes cold, damp weather
		Forgiveness
When balanced/imbalanced		Stability/greed

Ayurvedic practitioners use different methods to reestablish an individual's connection with nature and to realign imbalances. Allowing the body's natural forces to aid in healing is also important. Treatments are highly individualized and may involve changes to the diet, meditation, yoga, massage or exercise, herbal preparations, and lifestyle recommendations to address imbalances.

Calm digestion and elimination are often targeted in Ayurvedic care. Besides dietary changes, practitioners may also prescribe cleanses. Pancha karma is a type of stepwise cleanse that some followers of Ayurveda perform yearly for general health rejuvenation and prevention, as well as to foster spiritual release that will permit further spiritual growth.

The preparation phase involves the elimination of processed foods, stimulants such as coffee or caffeinated drinks, sweets, and often dairy products. Next, the diet is modified to one that is plant-based and plentiful in nutritious grains.

The final cleansing phase can involve fasting, juices, and different types of purges. Some of these methods may not be healthful for certain individuals and should be pursued with caution and under the dutiful care of an experienced practitioner.

Other Ayurvedic Practices

Treatments may include a combination of Ayurvedic remedies, most of which are botanical in origin. Some preparations may include mineral- or metal-based natural medicines, some of which can have the potential for toxicity. As with any unknown or uncertain formulation, be alert to possible safety concerns.

Turmeric and Curcumin

A relative of ginger, turmeric has been used for thousands of years in Indian cooking as a spice and is the main ingredient of curry, giving it its characteristic warm and intense yellow color. Dried turmeric powder contains curcumin, which is believed to confer many of turmeric's health benefits, including its antioxidant effects. People in India may routinely consume about 2 grams of turmeric daily, which provides about 100 milligrams of curcumin. In traditional Ayurvedic and Asian healing systems, turmeric has been used for wound antisepsis, inflammation, and cancer.

Modern research has demonstrated multiple ways that curcumin/ turmeric act on genes, enzymes, cell signaling, and other influencers of inflammation and cancer—including the spread of cancer (metastasis) beyond its primary site—and Alzheimer's disease. Small studies have shown benefits in mild and moderate ulcerative colitis, a form of inflammatory bowel disease.

Because curcumin and turmeric are some of the most promising and most actively studied natural substances being examined for a range of health effects, our understanding of these substances is expected to expand. Although turmeric and curcumin appear to be relatively safe in humans, even up to doses of 12 grams per day in one small human study, they are not as readily **bioavailable**, that is, they are not efficiently or easily absorbed or used by the body to achieve the desirable blood levels.

Some people may need to be especially cautious about using curcumin supplements that contain piperine, which is added to increase curcumin's bioavailability. Piperine may interfere with the metabolism of certain drugs, including phenytoin, an anti-seizure medicine, and others.

Ashwagandha

Also known as Indian ginseng or winter cherry, ashwagandha is a plant that is used in Ayurvedic herbology from its roots to the whole plant. It's formal Latin name is *Withania somnifera*. Rich in phytochemicals, ashwagandha is used traditionally as a tonic and for overall health, as well as for inflammation, stress, heart health, longevity, and cancer. Scientific studies have shown a variety of anti-cancer effects in the laboratory, although such effects have not yet been adequately studied in humans to justify firm conclusions. Preliminary studies have also looked at ashwagandha for diabetes and Parkinson's disease.

Ashwagandha supplements should list the amounts of active ingredients, known as **withanolides**, on the label. For root powders, look for a minimum of 0.3% withanolides and at least 1.5% withanolides in extracts. Powder formulas may be more stable than liquids. The doses used in human studies have ranged from about 1–6 grams for the root powder and 0.5–1.5 grams for the extract. A laboratory study in 2014 by independent supplement testing service ConsumerLab showed that many over-the-counter ashwagandha supplements lacked adequate active ingredients and/or exceeded the lab's established contamination levels for the heavy metals cadmium, arsenic, or lead.

Women who are pregnant or nursing as well as individuals with high blood pressure, diabetes, or thyroid conditions should opt for safety and reconsider using such supplements and, if at all, to do so under a knowledgeable health-care provider's care. Higher doses of ashwagandha may cause stomach upset or diarrhea.

Yoga

The practice of yoga, rooted in Ayurveda, is discussed in Chapter 7.

Finding an Ayurvedic Practitioner

Ayurvedic practitioners in the U.S. may come from a range of backgrounds, from yoga instructors to fully licensed medical doctors who have been trained in Ayurveda, perhaps in India. Stateside, Ayurveda is not a licensed medical profession as it is in many south Asian countries. However, some states are ahead of others in exploring and establishing standards of Ayurvedic care and licensure.

With its holistic approach that considers the mind, body, and spirit along with other facets of existence, Ayurveda offers pathways to health that include examining and modifying our habits, diet, activities, and emotional states—as well as our relationships with the natural world—to bring greater balance and peace to our lives.

HOMEOPATHY

Although homeopathy is relatively young as a whole system of care compared to Ayurveda or traditional Chinese medicine, it has become a popular form of alternative medicine. Increasingly, conventional medical practitioners are finding new uses for certain types of homeopathic care, illustrated by the use of the skin topical, arnica by dermatologists and surgeons to decrease pain or bruising. Lately, conventional practitioners have also considered homeopathic medicines for patients who desire antibiotics for situations in which antibiotics are unlikely to help and may instead contribute to increased antibiotic resistance.

Homeopathy was developed in the late 1800s by Samuel Hahnemann, a German physician and chemist. Experimenting with a Peruvian bark treatment for malaria on himself, colleagues, and subjects, Hahnemann developed the concept of "like cures like." Hahnemann came to believe that a substance that caused disease symptoms in healthy people might prove useful or curative in a person with similar symptoms. This concept forms the basis for the "law of similars," one of the main tenets of homeopathy. These theories stand in contrast to those of allopathic medicine, in which therapies are generally used to counter rather than weakly mimic the disease symptoms, regardless of their cause.

Like followers of homeopathy today, Hahnemann also believed in the body's innate ability to cure itself and to rid itself of disease. Hahnemann held that disturbances in the body's vital force were what led to illness and disease, which is somewhat similar to other belief systems that view prana or qi as essential to vitality and health.

The medicines of Hahnemann's day produced side effects, as occurs today with medicines of many types. Thus, he began experimenting with weaker concentrations or dilutions of medicines to cause the desired effect—cure or symptom relief—without producing the undesirable side effects. According to the chemical knowledge of his time, he also considered that he could influence certain molecular properties or strengths by subjecting them to different physical conditions. He developed the homeopathic belief that by shaking a solution very hard, termed **succussion**, a series of dilutions and succussions would fortify the medicine, allowing it to retain its strength to remedy illness, even if hardly an original molecule remained in the final solution, but not to cause undesired effects.

In line with the law of similars, according to homeopathic beliefs, lower doses of given remedies are viewed as actually more potent than more concentrated forms, which also differs from conventional medical practice beliefs. Rather, homeopaths maintain that minute amounts of homeopathic preparations are enough to trigger the body's innate ability to heal itself.

Mainstream medicine has been slow to accept that such heavily diluted homeopathic medicines are actually biologically active in the body. In fact, many studies have not proved a benefit to homeopathy beyond a placebo effect. However, the placebo effect is not insignificant and can be quite powerful, perhaps producing responses in up to 50% or more of certain people or in some situations or conditions. Homeopaths generally do not attribute homeopathic healing merely to placebo effects.

Homeopathic Treatments

As delivered by homeopaths, treatments are highly individualized and might involve combinations of botanicals, minerals, or other substances, ranging from crushed whole bees to potentially harmful plants such as poison ivy or belladonna. Treatments are generally not standardized among practitioners. One person's experience can be completely different in scope and methods from that of another person with the same or a similar condition.

Unlike most other dietary supplements, many homeopathic remedies are regulated by the FDA, although the FDA does not assess or test such medications for effectiveness or safety. Although they are heavily diluted in theory, homeopathic remedies may nonetheless contain significant amounts of active chemicals that could potentially provoke unwanted effects.

Most highly diluted homeopathic remedies on the market were considered nontoxic according to a 2007 study. However, if such remedies are likely to be ineffective and are being used in place of therapies that could probably help or cure a condition, the use of such seemingly harmless preparations could potentially delay healing or result in undesired complications.

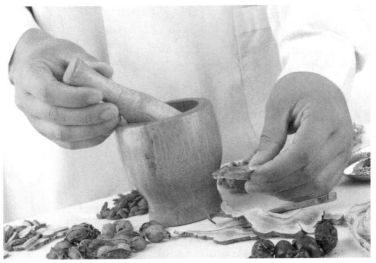

An herbalist prepares a customized preparation.

Consumers should also understand that many liquid homeopathic formulations might contain alcohol, sometimes at high levels. This feature should be factored in by individuals who should refrain from or avoid alcohol altogether, and by parents considering homeopathic remedies for their children. Many homeopathic medicines are made into sugar pellets that can be taken sublingually, or under the tongue.

Oscillococcinum® is a patented formulation that is one of the most commonly used homeopathic treatments and is used most often for flu or influenza. The dilution is made from an extract of duck liver and heart. Although a 2012 Cochrane systematic review of the evidence surrounding this preparation found no notable harmful effects of the medicine itself, the review also stated that there was not enough evidence of its effectiveness to support recommending its use in the prevention or treatment of influenza.

The Healing Crisis

In some situations, homeopaths may expect an individual to experience a temporary worsening of their condition or symptoms after beginning a homeopathic remedy. Termed "the healing crisis" or "homeopathic aggravation," this phase has not been readily explained by conventional medicine—if it does indeed exist as homeopaths maintain. Whether such a reaction is related to the homeopathic treatment itself or reflects the undertreatment or progression of the underlying disease or condition remains a matter of debate.

Uses of Homeopathy

Although homeopathy has been used to treat a range of disorders—from allergies to irritable bowel disorders—the evidence from large and well-conducted clinical trials in humans is weak to absent. Because many homeopathic treatments are themselves nontoxic, individuals may be interested in trying homeopathy. Notwithstanding, it should be appreciated that a treatment may not truly be considered nontoxic when a well-studied, safe, or established therapy that is available to cure or relieve the condition is not being used in favor of a homeopathic remedy.

Diseases or conditions for which homeopathy has been used include childhood diarrhea, allergies and rhinitis, colds and flu, pain syndromes or arthritis, bowel disorders, and dizziness or vertigo. For vertigo, homeopathic care seems to yield results that are similar to those obtained with mainstream medical care.

Finding a Homeopath

Before homeopathy clashed with the growing wave of science-based medical practice around the turn of the twentieth century, about a fifth of medical doctors in the U.S. incorporated homeopathic treatments in their practices. Today, standards and licensure requirements vary widely among the four main groups of homeopathic practitioners.

No testing, practice standards, or certification are required of **lay homeopaths**. **Professional homeopaths** typically receive about 1,000 training hours, yet—despite their name—they are not licensed health-care professionals. **Registered homeopathic medical assistants** receive about 300 hours of training but must work under the supervision of a licensed M.D. or D.O. **Licensed health-care professionals** such as naturopaths, chiropractors, and M.D.s may receive anywhere from about 200 to 1,000 training hours in homeopathy. Licensing and rules governing the scope of homeopathic practice vary from state to state.

NATUROPATHY

Founded as a comprehensive healing practice in the early 1900s, naturopathy is an integrated system of care that takes a holistic approach to the individual. Like some other whole systems of care, naturopathy embraces lifestyle approaches toward self-healing. These approaches can include nutrition, prevention, and the assistance of gentler remedies, including chiropractic, acupuncture, and homeopathy, among others. In a sense, naturopathy is an inclusive style of care that embraces many other healing methods, from the traditional to more modern approaches.

As with mainstream medicine, a central principle of naturopathic care is to do no harm—*primum non nocere*. Naturopaths aim to use methods that minimize side effects and to choose treatment methods that are considered less invasive or less potentially toxic than mainstream modalities. Naturopathy also emphasizes the power of nature and that of the body to heal the organism while also focusing on the underlying causes of disease and on removing obstacles to healing.

Along with prevention, naturopaths also value patient education. During a typical office visit, a naturopath will commonly invest a great deal of time with each patient, delving into his or her history to get a sense for the whole person and stressing preventive measures. Naturopaths value and forge partnership with their patients, aiding them in understanding their condition—as interpreted through the lens of naturopathy—and encouraging patients' involvement in their care.

Symptoms are viewed in naturopathy as indications of an imbalance. Rather than suppressing symptoms, naturopathic care is typically designed to address the cause of the imbalance so that healing can occur on all levels, from the physical to the spiritual and beyond.

To identify possible imbalances, naturopaths often rely on tests, including blood tests that some may consider to be of questionable reliability or validity. Today, such testing can include extensive genetic panels, even though many of the genetic associations that have been identified have not been fully fleshed out with respect to their ability to predict or confirm the presence or absence of a disease, condition, or risk factor.

Naturopaths may also pursue broad testing for exposure to environmental toxins and allergens to pinpoint the cause of symptoms, although—again—direct or reliable relationships between positive test results and actual illness or susceptibility have not been firmly established for many of these methods. Laboratories that perform esoteric testing using home-grown or nonstandard methods are receiving increased scrutiny along with consumer protection requests for accountability.

In general, naturopathic training may not provide the depth of expertise in molecular biology, clinical pathology, epidemiology, and statistics to fully support the critical use and interpretation of such tests, many of which have been used in humans for only a short time.

Such tests may not have been validated in large numbers of many different types of people to warrant the generalization of results, especially with regard to diagnosis or risk. False positive results are very common, meaning that a test result is positive, but the disease that the test is being used for is not actually present in that individual. Knowledge and reliability gaps between testing and interpretation are of particular concern with diploma naturopaths who have not fulfilled naturopathic doctor (N.D.) degree requirements at an accredited naturopathy school and naturopaths whose understanding of probabilities and laboratory medicine is limited.

Among the ways that naturopaths differ from most other integrative health-care professions is the unique requirement of homeopathy training for naturopaths. All naturopaths who complete the N.D. requirements at accredited naturopathy schools must complete homeopathic training that is recognized as meeting U.S. Department of Education standards. Naturopaths may also choose to receive additional training in acupuncture or minor surgery.

Uses of Naturopathy

Because a primary aim of naturopathy is to restore the body's ability to heal itself, people may seek naturopathic care for a variety of conditions, particularly chronic ones. Many individuals pursue naturopathy because of its focus on dietary and lifestyle factors, as well as its emphasis on overall wellness and prevention.

In the states and territories that have licensing or other regulations pertaining to the practice of naturopathy, naturopaths may function as primary care providers. Specialized naturopaths may also have practices that include pediatric or pregnant patients. In eight states, trained naturopaths may practice minor surgery, and in 11 states, they have certain prescription drug permissions to give injections of nutritionals, supplements, or even some drugs. Some naturopaths have parlayed their injection practice rights to delve into stem cell therapies.

As primary care providers, naturopaths see a wide range of illnesses and conditions. Naturopathic care may be especially appealing to people with many chronic diseases, dietary or nutritional issues, gastrointestinal disorders, allergies, diabetes, heart disease, or environmental concerns such as pollution or toxins.

In some practices or medical groups, naturopaths may participate in an integrative care model alongside M.D.s, D.O.s, and other mainstream health professionals. These naturopaths may practice integrative cancer care (oncology) or another type of specialized integrative care as part of a team that could also include specialists such as internists, rheumatologists, allergists, cardiologists, and even perhaps obstetrician/gynecologists.

Stem Cells: A New Chapter in Health and Healing?

Before our bodies developed their amazing and highly specialized complexity, first in the womb and then during growth, our earliest selves were composed of dividing cells that had the potential to become or differentiate into anything—from brain cells capable of sending chemical and electrical messages to bone cells destined to form our skeletons. Known as stem cells, these cells now form the basis of the billion-dollar global cell therapy industry. Because stem cells can be harvested from an individual—for example, from body fat—and injected back into that person's injured area, stem cell treatments are being viewed—and marketed—as natural and less risky than other therapies.

Practitioners interested in this type of regenerative medicine or tissue engineering have been flocking to stem cell treatments for a variety of pain disorders, immune conditions, and degenerative diseases. Despite its roots in cell engineering and ultramodern technology, some naturopaths are promoting stem cells as natural alternatives for aging skin and as possible alternatives to orthopedic and other types of surgery—even face-lifts.

Taken altogether, the booming interest in cell therapies, the perception that they are harmless and natural alternative therapies, the lack of regulation, and massive investments worldwide have combined to create a type of "Wild West" in the cell therapy field. There has been no proof that these treatments are ready for the open market or that they work as intended for all the conditions for which they are being used. In many cases, it is unclear whether any stem cells are being infused at all. The cell therapy frenzy has also spawned a new category of supplements that claim to activate or increase a person's stem cells for conditions ranging from Alzheimer's to wrinkles. Although the promise of cell therapies is great, to date these claims and such uses remain unproven, with an unknown potential for harm.

Increasingly, naturopaths and other integrative and alternative practitioners are embracing regenerative medicine, typified by stem cell treatments and **prolotherapy**, a special type of injection that uses an irritating substance in an attempt to heal injured tissues such as joints and ligaments. Although this method has been used for more than a century, the evidence for its benefits in conditions that range from back pain to knee osteoarthritis and a variety of sports injuries remains weak and inconclusive for most conditions.

Future studies should help determine whether prolotherapy will prove to be effective, particularly for chronic tendon problems such as tennis elbow and Achilles pain, as well as for back pain and knee arthritis, for which limited studies have suggested that the therapy may hold promise.

Finding a Naturopath

Use the link at the end of this chapter for the American Association of Naturopathic Physicians to help find a naturopath who has graduated from an accredited school of naturopathy. See Chapter 2 for more information about the growing number of states with licensing requirements for naturopaths.

CHIROPRACTIC

Founded in 1895 by Daniel David Palmer, an Iowa schoolteacher who was interested in magnetic healing, chiropractic is based on the belief that the body possesses the innate power to heal itself. Palmer had seen a man who reportedly became deaf after an incident that caused an abnormal formation to develop in his back area. Thinking that perhaps the man's spinal deformity had led to his deafness, Palmer sought to reverse his hearing loss by manipulating his spine. After the man was said to have regained his hearing following Palmer's manipulation, Palmer developed his theory of chiropractic by which he considered health and disease as states that could be influenced by the alignment of the spine.

Today, there are an estimated 75,000 chiropractors in the U.S. Unlike naturopaths, chiropractors are licensed in all 50 states.

Chiropractors seek to investigate and address structural imbalances that have led to a condition or disease such as altered spinal alignment, flexibility, and posture, as well as other factors, including nutrition, lifestyle, stress, and others. Thus, chiropractic care is holistic and highly centered on the individual patient. As a result, chiropractic interviews may be lengthy, especially when the client is seen for the first time.

The goals of chiropractic care are not only to relieve symptoms but also to identify and address other factors that might require correction or modification to promote optimal health and wellness. These latter goals may involve acupuncture, bodywork or mind-body therapies, nutrition, and supplements, among others.

Most chiropractors primarily use physical methods in the care of their patients. Manual methods such as spinal or joint manipulation, stretching, and therapeutic massage are common. Other therapies such as ultrasound, electrotherapy, or hydrotherapy may also be used, which focus the energy of sound waves, electric current, or water, respectively, on the ailing part or to the body in general. Chiropractors are increasingly experimenting with lower-force techniques, typically using devices or special equipment.

Better Healing Through Technology: Low-Level Laser (Light) Therapy

Based on research by the National Aeronautics and Space Administration, low-level laser therapy, also known as low-level light therapy (LLLT), was introduced in 1967. The use of such devices by qualified professionals was cleared by the FDA in 2003 as an add-on therapy for temporary pain relief. In some states, a prescription is required. Today, it has become a widely adopted therapy used by chiropractors and other health professionals ranging from physical therapists and sports medicine physicians to dermatologists, cardiologists, and wound healing specialists such as vascular and plastic surgeons. Neurologists are also interested in LLLT for its possible benefit in stroke recovery.

The idea behind LLLT is that the energy delivered by such devices is able to deeply penetrate into damaged tissues, wherein it may spur or accelerate healing, increase blood supply, and decrease pain or inflammation. The biology of tissue reaction to LLLT is very complex, and the optimal use of this therapy is far from being completely understood. For example, it is still unclear whether continuous or pulsed light is better, and for which condition or situation. The optimal amount of LLLT time, the interval, the wavelength, and different factors related to the intensity of the treatment also have not been precisely determined in the variety of conditions for which LLLT is being used. LLLT should not be used near the eyes, in pregnant women, or for areas of the body where the skin might have suspicious or precancerous lesions because of safety concerns. The long-term effects of LLLT are also unknown.

The growing list of conditions for which LLLT is being used includes various types of musculoskeletal and nerve pain, temporomandibular disorders (TMJ) and carpal tunnel pain, hair loss, and problems related to healing or lymphatic drainage, among others. Many insurance companies and government insurers consider LLLT largely experimental and do not pay for such services, which can sometimes involve a commitment to 30 sessions at considerable expense and questionable justification.

Consider getting a second opinion about LLLT therapy from someone familiar with your specific condition to help determine if it might be worth pursuing as an add-on therapy. Following the release of new guidelines regarding LLLT in cancer patients who could develop mouth lesions as a result of cancer therapy, the uses for LLLT appear poised to expand and to evolve in the coming years.

Special pressure techniques known as "adjustments" may be applied to manipulate certain joints. Typically performed with a rapid but highly specific thrust of the hand and arm, adjustments are the hallmark of chiropractic practice.

Uses of Chiropractic

Most people seek out chiropractic care for physical ailments or pain involving the musculoskeletal system of bones and joints. Among these, back and neck pain are the most common conditions, along with various sports-related injuries.

Besides musculoskeletal problems, individuals may seek chiropractic care for other ailments including headaches, allergies, hormonal problems, gastrointestinal disturbances, chronic fatigue disorders, insomnia, high blood pressure, and other conditions treated by primary care providers. Therapies might include different types of manual therapies, nutritional interventions, counseling, acupuncture, and supplements.

Frequently, a chiropractic care program demands multiple therapeutic sessions, perhaps as many as 30, averaging 17 visits per year in one study. Known as extended or maintenance care, such visits are considered an unnecessary service by Medicare and are not reimbursed. The benefits of maintenance care to patients remain in question.

Evidence for the effectiveness of chiropractic manipulation is strongest for routine back pain—whether acute or recent, somewhat recent (subacute), or longer term (chronic). Certain types of neck pain that were not caused by a traumatic incident such as a car accident or fall may also be helped by chiropractic manipulation. Some evidence also supports the value of chiropractic manipulation for chronic headaches.

Chiropractic care may also benefit older adults with chronic pain conditions; however, caution should always be used in any individual with weak or brittle bones, bleeding disorders, nerve problems such as numbness and tingling, surgical implants or prior surgery, serious underlying health problems, prior stroke or blood vessel disease, or cancer.

Finding a Chiropractor

Chiropractors may use physical examination, a series of questions, and diagnostic tests to arrive at a diagnosis and to develop a treatment plan. Chiropractors may also refer their patients to other health-care professionals, including conventional medical doctors, when necessary. Ask a trusted health-care professional for names of chiropractors to whom they regularly refer patients and with whom they have had a successful professional relationship.

Like naturopaths, some chiropractors are permitted to perform minor surgery, although this is limited to only a few states. In New Mexico, chiropractors may have limited prescription rights. Some chiropractors are involved in obstetrical care depending on the state's regulations and the individual chiropractor's training and licensure. Certain states offer chiropractors a broad range of practice options, whereas other states are more restrictive as to what a chiropractor may or may not do.

If your interest in chiropractic care is more specialized, understand that after graduating from chiropractic colleges, chiropractors may receive additional training or certification in diagnostic imaging, pediatrics, sports injuries, nutrition, and other fields. Increasingly, chiropractors are also involved in research.

Use the link for the American Chiropractic Association at the end of this chapter and the additional information in Chapter 2 to find out more about locating a qualified chiropractic practitioner in your state.

WHERE TO LEARN MORE

National Ayurvedic Medical Association: *www.ayurvedanama.org*

North American Society of Homeopaths: *www.homeopathy.org*

American Association of Naturopathic Physicians: *www.naturopathic.org*

American Chiropractic Association: *www.acatoday.org*

The World Health Organization's 2014–2023 Traditional Medicine Strategy, available in Arabic, Chinese, English, French, Russian, and Spanish: *http://www.who.int/medicines/publications/traditional/trm_strategy14_23/en/*

11

Special Topics

THIS CHAPTER INVITES YOU TO DELVE DEEPER INTO A FEW SPECIAL TOPICS THAT don't fall neatly into other sections of this book. As with the other information presented, new knowledge in these areas is growing rapidly. Tap into the sources listed at the end of this chapter and additional information given throughout the book for the latest findings, and discuss them with your health-care team.

DETOXIFICATION/CLEANSING

During the normal process of cellular events throughout our body, waste products are formed and later cleared or eliminated from the body. When systems or organisms are functioning normally, these waste products are mostly excreted through the liver and kidney but also through the lungs, skin, lymphatic system, and the gastrointestinal tract.

Thoughts and behaviors that could be considered as toxic can also be released or neutralized by the brain, as when we successfully cope with a stressful situation or overcome an unreasonable fear or anxiety.

When or if waste products, toxins, or metabolites are allowed to build up in the body or mind, as occurs in many disease states, harmful consequences can follow.

Despite a great deal of evidence to the contrary, many people seek to kick-start or to accelerate the body's detoxification. Others may occasionally or regularly purge their system as part of a general health tune-up or as part of a cleansing or purification process.

Detoxification is a general term and can mean different things to different people. To some, detoxification is a necessity of modern living, brought on by the perceived need to rid the body of substances that are believed to have been absorbed or taken in from the environment. These environmental concerns can involve fears or concerns about plastic residues, chemical pollutants, invisible energy forms such as radiation, and even exposure to cleaners and chemicals used in everyday life.

As the list of agents to which we are exposed in the course of a typical day anywhere in the world today grows, people concerned about healthy living would understandably wish to limit or eliminate their exposure to potentially damaging substances. We do, after all, live in a fossil-fueled chemical world.

Nevertheless, whereas some may view detoxification as a required wellness ritual that is restorative and invigorating, physical detoxification can seem unappealing or unnecessary to others.

Periodic detoxifications through cleansing, fasting, and/or diet are often pursued in Ayurveda, traditional Chinese medicine, and other traditional healing methods. Detoxification is also stressed with many fad or elimination diets, which often target a food or food component considered as "toxic," although such potential harm may be exaggerated or undeserved, or it may only apply to a small fraction of the population. A recent example is the rejection of gluten-containing foods including nourishing whole grains—which, although symptom triggers for the minority of people with true celiac disease, can safely be part of a healthful diet for most people.

Besides physical detoxification, mental detoxification can be considered when negative thought processes, chronically poor choices, behaviors that are not life-enhancing or well-adapted, an inability to release from the past, limited resilience, excessive cynicism, or other unhealthy behaviors are a concern. Substance abuse can also be approached with both physical and mental detoxification, both of which are best pursued under the care of a competent integrative health professional.

Detox Targets

These are a few of the targets of different detoxification regimens.

Environmental: Pollutants, heavy metals, allergens.

Mental/behavioral: Addictions, stress, negative behaviors and thoughts.

Nonnutritive food-like substances (so-called antinutrients): Transfats, high-fructose corn syrup, and processed foods.

Internal: Metabolites and by-products of internal processes that maintain us or those related to medications, both prescription and over-the-counter.

Infectious: Microbes, parasites, and viruses.

Finding a Detoxification Program for Your Needs

Many different types of detox therapies are available. Finding your method of choice will depend on your reasons for seeking detoxification and your overall health. Also important is your acceptance of or tolerance for certain detoxification techniques. Work with a provider who understands your health history, your current medical or psychological issues, and your goals to arrive at a plan that is reasonable, safe, and effective.

Typically, a detoxification program includes all or some of the following:

- Nutritional therapy, changes, or fasting.
- Physical activity, whether strenuous or relaxing.
- Inward focus, as with meditation, mind-body practices, or breathing exercises.
- Touch therapy such as massage or another bodywork technique.

Some regimens also include some type of purge, sometimes through profuse sweating, enemas, or colonics. The benefit of such therapies remains in doubt. Moreover, certain methods could be risky, unpleasant, or dehydrating for some people.

Be sure to discuss a detoxification program that you are considering with your health-care provider. Because you may be asked to stop taking prescription medicines during a detox program, symptoms may develop that could need attention. Certain aspects of different detoxification programs, such as prolonged fasting, pared-down diets, or intestinal cleansing, may not be right for you.

Remember not to overlook other ways that toxic influences may have crept into daily life and from which relief would be therapeutic. For example, consider taking a break from long mindless sessions in front of electronics or from packaged "entertainment" involving violence, cruelty, or other negative behaviors across all media. Consider dialing back other obsessive behaviors or energy related to celebrity culture, narcissism, or chronic materialism that offer little value, relevance, or betterment to our overall existence. Take a break from nonnurturing friends or situations, gossip, chronic hostility, and other activities that are not life enhancing.

Detox mentally, physically, and spiritually by realigning how you use precious time. Use the hours salvaged from TV watching or other time drains to instead engage with learning, loved ones, and family. Exalt in that reclaimed time for active living, whether by participating in a healthful physical activity, a beloved hobby or a new interest that offers some element of growth, inner peace, and satisfaction.

Not only will such a cleanse improve overall health and metabolism, but it may also boost overall immune status, as has been shown for exercise. Gather a renewed sense of connectedness and physical and psychosocial well-being by engaging in more regular physical activity and by being more involved in meaningful social, personal, or spiritual endeavors.

Is Screen Time Killing You?

Recent studies from Europe and Australia have produced alarming statistics on TV viewing time and death rates from all causes, not just heart disease. Four or more hours of average daily TV viewing nearly doubled the risk of dying of any cause and tripled the chances of a cardiovascular death compared to people who watched less than two hours per day, according to an Australian study of nearly 9,000 adults aged 25 or older. (The average American watches about five hours of television daily.) The risk of early death remained higher even in TV watchers who exercised regularly, and these risks increased with every additional hour spent watching TV. The study participants and controls were matched for age, weight, and other factors. The investigators thought that these disturbing findings might be explained by prolonged periods spent sitting still. Screen time that also involves disengagement or unhealthy eating or drinking can heighten this health nightmare—one that apparently may also be deadly yet is quite preventable.

CHELATION

Medical chelation is a chemical method used to extract heavy metals such as lead, cadmium, mercury, and others from the bloodstream. The procedure usually involves the use of an injection form of EDTA, a chemical that binds these metals. In cases of heavy metal poisoning or overexposure, chelation is an accepted method used to remove such toxic substances.

Beyond such uses, various practitioners—including anti-aging advocates—have proposed chelation therapy for other conditions. Chelation has been used and promoted for heart disease—specifically as a nonsurgical method to reverse atherosclerosis, or hardening of the arteries, in which cholesterol and calcium deposits lodge and accumulate within the artery wall. Certain autoimmune diseases such as lupus and scleroderma have also been targets for chelation therapy, as have children with autism spectrum disorders.

Is there evidence to support these other uses of chelation beyond heavy metal poisoning? The short answer appears to be no.

Although advocates for chelation have claimed to have successfully treated hundreds of thousands or millions of people with this method, there is nearly a complete absence of well-controlled studies in the literature to demonstrate that this method works as intended or that its results are significantly better than those obtained with conventional care or placebo. Although chelation has been criticized as being one of the biggest consumer health frauds, a 2013 study in the *Journal of the American Medical Association* involving about 1,700 people who had heart attacks showed that the possible slight positive benefits of chelation on blood vessel biology deserve further investigation.

ENVIRONMENTAL HEALTH

Living a clean life, inside and out, can be a challenge in a world dependent on fossil fuels. We come into contact with a daily buffet of chemicals in our lives, from our morning personal care routines to dreaded commutes in exhaust-spewing bumper-to-bumper traffic.

Ways to Create Healthier Indoor Living

- Commit to smoke-free living, including second- and third-hand smoke.
- Maintain a clean, well-ventilated, and dust-free home, and change air filters often.
- Use only cold water for drinking, rinsing produce, and food preparation.
- Maintain heaters, chimneys, furnaces, and fireplaces to avoid carbon monoxide exposure, and install a monitoring device—especially in colder climates.
- Test your home for radon levels and take action if there are 4 picocuries per liter of air or more.
- Use nontoxic cleaners whenever possible, and always use them with good ventilation.
- Choose greener options for flooring, furniture, tableware, clothing, nourishment, personal care, and accessories.
- Learn to cook using more nutrient-preserving and energy-efficient techniques such as pressure cooking.
- Wipe your feet or shoes when reentering your home from outside.
- Wash your hands well with soap and warm water before touching indoor objects after being at work or outside.
- Commit to saving the precious resources of water and energy at every opportunity.

Nevertheless, outside of picking up stakes and moving to an eco-sustainable fantasy island, we can endeavor to commit to basic practices, if not more, to improve the quality of our environmental health. It may be more effective to influence some of the factors that govern our indoor lives, where we spend much—if not most—of our time on this planet, including the one-third of our lives spent sleeping.

GENETICS

Personalized medicine, once a dream, is rapidly becoming a reality. The success of the Human Genome Project has had far-reaching effects on our understanding of our genetic makeup.

We already know that many diseases and cancers result from changes or mutations of the DNA that make up our genes. We are now just beginning to examine the ways in which we might be able to influence how our genes behave through lifestyle changes and, so it is hoped, to have greater control over our health. Although somewhat oversimplified and inaccurate, some have referred to these early findings as "changing our DNA," whether through exercise, diet changes, stress management, or other means.

One way to understand these modifications of our gene activity, known as **epigenetics** and **epigenomics** (see sidebar), is to consider them together as similar to great software that allows you to get many more things out of your computer without changing your hardware or getting a new computer—or to do them faster, more efficiently, or better.

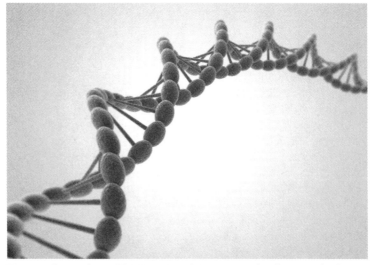

Humans have about 20,000 to 25,000 genes made of DNA, which store messages or recipes that govern how we look, how our bodies function, and our health.

Learning the New Language of Genetics

To understand what all the talk about genes and genetics is all about, get familiar with the language of this exciting field.

DNA
Deoxyribonucleic acid, a double-stranded helix of coded hereditary information mostly stored inside the nucleus of a cell in tightly packaged structures (like a ball of string) called chromosomes.

Genes
Basic hereditary units made of DNA that contain instructions for making proteins that guide or signal our growth and health and that occur in pairs—one inherited from each parent, like beads on a string.

Genetics
The study of heredity, often as relates to single genes.

Epigenetics
The study of modifications to our DNA and genes that do not involve changes of the genetic code itself but that may affect the activity, silencing, or expression of a gene.

Epigenomics
The study of changeable chemical tags that mark the genome and help determine which genes are active or how they are to function or behave; the chemical tags of the epigenome may be related to what we eat, drugs, and other factors or exposures in the environment.

Chromosome
Tightly wound strings of genes within the nucleus, the control center of cells; humans have 23 pairs of chromosomes, with one from each pair donated by each parent.

Genome
The total DNA of an organism, including all of its genes.

Genomics
The study or mapping of genes and their function(s), often in groups or altogether to study their combined influence (for example, on growth or health).

Human Genome Project
An international research effort begun in 1990 to map the entire human genome and the genes contained; completed (ahead of schedule) in 2003.

Can You Really Change Your DNA?

Unlike a gene or chromosome, both of which have an actual structure, the epigenome is a constellation of factors that can influence or modify the way a gene behaves. For example, chemical tags known as methyl groups can be added to or removed from your DNA depending on what you eat or drink, medications, physical activity, your stress levels, or even whether or not you smoke.

This **methylation** can turn a gene on or off, or perhaps cause cells to grow or not grow. Should epigenetic factors cause cells to grow at the wrong time or at the wrong pace, certain cancers may develop.

Our understanding of the epigenome is growing, but it remains fairly basic and preliminary. Although the epigenome remains to be fully explained, we already know that lifestyle factors can indeed have powerful effects on our health. We can strive to maximize healthful lifestyle choices, regardless of whether they are tested by genetic methods. Be wary of practitioners or products offering easy answers to methylation and this complex, incompletely understood area of specialized science. Question whether tests aimed at determining your genetic risks, often coupled with more tests or the purchase of particular nutritional supplements or expensive treatments, are indeed serving your best interest.

Genetic Testing: Ready for Prime Time?

A variety of tests have accompanied the explosion in our genetic knowledge. Testing that can reliably forecast our risk for macular degeneration in adults or Type I diabetes are now joined by tests whose reliability may be hardly better than a coin toss, as with certain tests for Alzheimer's risk, heart disease (as a function of certain vitamin metabolism genes), or other common conditions. Yet, despite these performance gaps, tests are in demand and testing is on the rise.

Some genetic tests have been available directly to consumers, and others are available to health-care practitioners, who are expected to competently and responsibly order, review, interpret, and discuss such results with their patients. However, not all providers who order such tests have been adequately trained or are prepared to do so.

Just because a test exists doesn't necessarily mean that the test is good or valid, or that the results apply to people of your race, age, condition, or ethnic background. The claims surrounding some genetic tests have made it difficult to interpret the value of this new information or whether the results can truly be applied or personalized to that particular individual.

Consider the following points when approaching a decision about whether to have genetic testing:

- Is the test ready for prime time—that is, is the test or panel a good predictor of the disease in question? Most tests for common diseases have not proved to be very good predictors of risk or that they are better than current screening methods (at least not yet).
- Do you feel prepared to cope with results that may be discouraging? If you do not, reconsider having the test at all or discuss your concerns further with your practitioner before proceeding.
- How committed are you to taking action or changing your behavior in light of the test results? Studies of consumer-driven testing have shown that such testing hasn't helped motivate individuals into making lifestyle changes. When studied, most smokers continued to smoke, regardless of such test results. Consider your own resistance or openness to change.
- Have you begun or been open to addressing any known risk factors due to your family history? Right now, that history is about as informative as most genetic test results.

Harnessing the information encoded in our genes and epigenomes promises to open up new avenues toward personalized health care. In time, these new paths may help us achieve greater control over our health—provided that we are motivated and willing to make the choices or changes necessary. At present, however, this is a rapidly evolving area of inquiry with a great deal of ground left to cover. Questions far outnumber firm answers thus far, at least outside of targeted cancer therapies or already known risk factors.

Before embarking on costly or esoteric genetic testing that could be coupled with a new regimen of supplements or office visits involving further dubious testing, reconsider whether you are doing all you can to maximize your health and to address any known issues in your family history. Redouble your efforts by concentrating on these simple yet proven methods to live a healthier life:

- Avoid tobacco in all forms.
- Maintain a healthy weight, and pay attention to excess weight around your midsection.
- Eat a healthy diet, and increase your intake of plant-based foods.
- Get plenty of physical activity regularly, including strength training and aerobic fitness.
- Limit sit-down periods or sedentary behaviors.
- Stay connected, optimistic, and mentally challenged.

- Perform attitude and engagement tune-ups regularly, and refresh as needed.
- Live a loving life.

The evidence for the benefits of these behaviors is very strong. A recent study of nearly 70,000 women who were followed for 20 years showed that almost three-quarters of all cases of heart disease—and nearly half of all cases of diabetes, high blood pressure, and high cholesterol or triglycerides—could be avoided by adopting the first five of the behaviors above, along with drinking no more than one alcoholic drink per day. It's doubtful whether treatments designed around genetic testing or any currently available therapy—conventional, alternative, or integrative—can top that.

CANCER

With cancer survivorship on the rise, more people living with cancer are turning to integrative methods, both during their cancer care and during survivorship. As of early 2014, nearly 15 million Americans with a history of cancer were alive, with most having passed the five-year mark since their cancer diagnosis.

Many of the side effects of cancer and its treatment can be successfully managed with the help of integrative care methods. Not surprisingly, cancer patients, survivors, and their families are asking about and looking to such therapies for symptom relief.

Most people with cancer don't expect to be cured by integrative methods. Rather, the most common reasons for seeking out integrative cancer care include getting relief from symptoms or side effects of cancer or its treatment along with improving overall quality of life and wellness. Another common reason people seek integrative oncology care is to satisfy the wish or need to have some control over their illness and their overall health status, as well as perhaps to boost their immune system.

Besides the usual recommendations for maintaining health during cancer care and beyond (namely, getting enough exercise; maintaining nurturing support systems; and following a healthy diet rich in fruits, vegetables, and whole grains and low in processed and red meat, fat, and simple sugars), cancer specialists and cancer patients themselves may also be interested in other integrative therapies. These include mind-body relaxation methods, acupuncture, certain supplements, gentle manual methods, and movement therapies such as tai chi.

New Opportunities: Integrative Care for Common Side Effects of Cancer and Cancer Treatments

Consult the Method Finder in Chapter 14 and other chapters in this book to explore with your health-care provider whether integrative care may be useful for these and other side effects of cancer or cancer treatments.

Thinning of the bones (osteoporosis)
Damage to the heart (cardiotoxicity)
Mental changes ("chemo brain," memory problems, and others)
Anxiety and fear
Depression
Fatigue
Infertility (after certain types of treatments)
Pain
Arm swelling (after breast surgery)
Breathing, nerve, or muscle problems
Loss of appetite, weight loss
Sexual problems
Lowering of immunity

Dietary Supplements and Cancer Care

Up to 90% of patients with cancer use dietary supplements, often by their own choice and frequently without informing their health-care team. Although generally not taken with the expectation of cure, the use of some of these supplements in particular can cause interactions with drugs used during cancer care or survivorship. Moreover, some supplements may have potentially harmful side effects on organs that may have been damaged by chemotheraphy or radiation therapy, or on organs that are at higher risk of becoming injured by certain supplement doses or chemicals.

In 2013, a group of doctors within the Society of Integrative Oncology published a list of 10 supplements that cancer patients and their doctors may wish to explore and discuss together. The landmark article also provided helpful information on known side effects and concerns, along with the doses that appeared to be useful at that time. This information, and the groundbreaking activities of that group, is certain to be revisited and revised in the future as our knowledge of this important aspect of cancer care and survivorship grows.

Dietary Supplements in Cancer Care*

Supplement	Actions or Target	Cautions or Side Effects	Amount Studied
Curcumin	Tumor inhibition; may enhance effects of chemotheraphy or radiation therapy	Gastrointestinal (GI) symptoms (high doses); use caution with gallbladder disease	500–3,000 mg
Glutamine	For chemo-induced GI tract effects or neuropathy	Use caution with liver or kidney disease or the use of anti-seizure drugs	5–30 g per day
Vitamin D	Anti-tumor effects	Safe overall	Dose according to vitamin D levels
Maitake mushrooms	Anti-tumor, immune-boosting effects	Safe overall; caution with diabetes or blood-thinning drugs and certain immune states or tumors	Variable
Fish oil (omega-3 fatty acids)	Anti-tumor or anti-inflammatory effects	Mild GI effects; possible bleeding risk	2–3 g per day
Green tea	Anti-tumor effects	Safe in beverage form with moderate intake; possible interactions with anti-clotting drugs and some chemotherapy	~ 3 cups per day
Milk thistle	Liver protection	Possible laxative effect; may increase tamoxifen levels	200–400 mg per day
Astragalus	Immune effects	Overall well tolerated; may interact with some chemotherapy or immune-suppressant drugs	Variable
Melatonin	Anti-tumor effects	Safe overall; may have interactions with blood sugar or with anti-clotting and other drugs and foods	Variable
Probiotics	Immune and intestinal anti-toxic effects	Safe overall; caution with iron supplement use	Variable

Source: Adapted with permission from Frenkel, M., and Sierpina, V., "The Use of Dietary Supplements in Oncology" in *Current Oncology Reports*, September 2014.

*Amounts used in individual care may vary; consult your health-care team before using these or any other dietary supplements in cancer care.

Cancer Care and Antioxidants

The use of antioxidant supplements in cancer care is controversial. Because antioxidants can potentially help reverse or fight damage produced by tumor cells, it could seem that more antioxidants, in the form of supplements, would be better. Studies show that this may not always be the case. We are learning that there is more to the balance between antioxidants and reactive oxygen species than can be solved by merely bathing cancer cells with more antioxidants from supplements.

In fact, some recent studies have suggested that malignant cells possess unique ways to get around hostile chemical environments and may instead take advantage of an antioxidant-rich microenvironment. This may help explain why it appears that supplementation with two nutrients, vitamin E and beta-carotene, may actually increase cancer risk in certain people.

The recommendations regarding the use of antioxidants in cancer care are still in flux. While it appears safe and overall preferable for cancer patients and survivors to consume diets that are naturally rich in antioxidants, the question of supplementation is under debate, with strong advocates on each side of the equation.

Radiation oncologists and medical oncologists who administer anti-cancer drugs may be adamant about their patients not using any dietary supplements beyond a regular-strength multivitamin while they are undergoing radiation or chemotherapy. Yet, some integrative oncologists express confidence regarding the beneficial potential of certain antioxidants in cancer care.

As with other aspects of cancer and general health care, talk this over with your care team to decide the best path for you. Also, consider a consultation with an integrative oncologist if you wish to explore these and other integrative methods in your cancer care and survivorship.

WHERE TO LEARN MORE

Society for Integrative Oncology: *www.integrativeonc.org*

National Human Genome Research Institute: *www.genome.gov*

American Association for Clinical Chemistry, a collaborative resource on laboratory testing: *www.labtestsonline.org*

National Center for Environmental Health, Centers for Disease Control and Prevention: *www.cdc.gov/nceh/*

Clinical trial opportunities for cancer and a variety of conditions and methods, including genetic and genomic studies, chelation, and detoxification: *www.clinicaltrials.gov*

12

Self-Care and Prevention

UILDING A CULTURE OF HEALTH BEGINS WITH INDIVIDUAL EFFORTS. ALTHOUGH we look to institutions such as state-of-the-art health centers and the health industry to aid us when we get sick, staying healthy for as long as possible begins with individual efforts toward self-care and prevention throughout daily life.

In this chapter, self-care and prevention are brought into focus. Self-care not only involves your own attempts to foster and maintain health but also includes preventive efforts that help safeguard you from other hazards in life—from accidents to preventable illnesses.

Attitudes toward self-care, empowerment, and prevention will influence which strategies seem right or natural for you and which might require greater focus or new habit-building behaviors. Wherever you fall on that spectrum, this chapter offers healing ways to healthier, more sustainable living.

COMPLEX SOLUTIONS, SIMPLE TRUTHS

A buffet of health news arrives in our inboxes and doorsteps daily. The latest facts and factoids send us scurrying to the Internet, our health-care providers, or our favorite media health star for more information. Studies, statistics, and testimonials can sometimes rivet our attention, perhaps sidestepping the fact that the long-term effectiveness and the side effects of such remedies are often unknown or are preliminary at best.

Lost in this complex decision-making about new treatments that require us to weigh incomplete facts and unknowns are a few simple facts that have reliably been shown to help maintain and improve health as well as longevity. Many long-term studies by respected groups around the world, including the Centers for Disease Control, the World Health Organization, and the American Heart Association, have shown that certain core behaviors are associated with longer, healthier living:

- Avoiding or quitting tobacco use.
- Getting regular exercise.
- Eating a healthy diet.
- Limiting alcohol.
- Maintaining a normal body mass index (BMI, a measurement of an appropriate weight for your height).

Along with this basic list are other habits or behaviors that must not be discounted, such as always wearing your seat belt, taking advantage of available preventive care, and following the recommended immunization schedule for your age group.

As promising as many of the therapies discussed in this book are, following the simple guidelines above can provide a solid foundation for health and wellness.

Leading Causes of Death in the United States

According to the CDC, the top five leading causes of death in the U.S. are:

1. Heart disease
2. Cancer
3. Chronic lower respiratory diseases
4. Stroke
5. Unintentional injuries (including accidents, motorized vehicle incidents, overdoses, and suicides)

Most of these are lifestyle related and most are, you guessed it, preventable.

THE POWER OF PREVENTION

Most people would agree that prevention is a good thing. After all, how can you be opposed to preventing pain, disability, and early or avoidable death? Too often, however, the praise of prevention is more lip service than a truly purposeful and effective preventive effort. Prevention is, after all, an effort.

Why is this? Why is prevention, which seems like such a no-brainer, so difficult to pursue or achieve? Why is the road to prevention, something that most people seem ready to embrace, littered with roadblocks and obstacles?

Part of the answer lies with the fact that even when prevention works as designed and expected, its success is invisible. Take the case of polio, for example. This devastating disease is caused by a virus that attacks the nervous system, causing paralysis and even death. Polio epidemics swept across the U.S. and the world during the last century. In 1952, the number of polio cases peaked stateside, affecting nearly 60,000 children in that year alone—killing 3,000 kids and leaving thousands more paralyzed for life. Parents lived in fear that polio would claim their children, a fear that drove public swimming pools to close. Sick and paralyzed children were cared for in devices known as iron lungs when they were unable to breathe on their own. Worldwide, the toll was even greater.

Polio even affected President Franklin D. Roosevelt, who contracted the dreaded disease a few years before he became president. Both Presidents Roosevelt and Harry Truman made the prevention of polio a priority, and by 1955, a widespread vaccination effort was underway. By 1979, the U.S. was a polio-free nation, and the disease that had implanted terror in parents' hearts had now been prevented, becoming virtually invisible—especially to future generations.

Despite the success of this monumental preventive effort, a subsequent generation took the absence of vaccine-preventable diseases for granted. For some diseases, decreased rates of vaccination have led to the reemergence of potentially fatal diseases such as measles, pertussis (whooping cough), and, sadly—in some parts of the world—polio itself.

Similarly, the lung cancers that are prevented by stopping smoking are not seen, just as the ravages of diabetes that fail to occur in people who learn to control their blood sugar—or who prevent the development of diabetes in the first place—are invisible complications, prevented from ever happening.

Besides invisibility and its lack of drama, prevention can be difficult. Prevention often involves persistent commitment or change. Quitting smoking presents a tough task for smokers, and successful quitting typically involves at least five or six unsuccessful attempts. Dieters also know how difficult it can be to lose excess weight, even those pesky five to 10 pounds.

Prevention is sometimes viewed as an uphill battle in this age of instant rewards, in part because preventive behaviors typically require long periods of time before the benefits are reaped. While most vaccines offer fairly short-term results in terms of immunity to a disease, many other preventive behaviors require the prevention-minded to follow a consistent course of action (for example, eating right or always wearing a seat belt) or inaction (as in eliminating tobacco) over years and often decades.

Sadly, the current health system is far more nimble at intervention than prevention. Thus, it becomes even more important for individuals who care about and who seek to direct their own health to embrace prevention wherever and whenever possible.

NUTRITION

Year-round, books about eating and dieting dominate the bestseller list, especially after the New Year. Many of these books make eating seem pretty complicated or confusing. Often, the diets that are touted are fabricated eating plans and are not living diets at all. That is, they are not diets or ways of eating that people follow and have followed over time as part of normal living, such as the Mediterranean diet.

Despite all the multimedia static about diet, it is possible to make sense out of eating well by taking into account a few facts, concepts, and goals.

First, it's important to realize that developing healthier eating habits doesn't have to be burdensome or overwhelming. True, it can be difficult to break out of lifelong habits or family traditions that may have pre-seasoned your palate to desire sweet, salty, or otherwise unhealthy foods. It is also true that most of us will never have the skills and creativity of television and restaurant chefs, not to mention those helpful sous chefs standing by.

For most of us, learning to eat healthier will require new skill sets. Learning to make better choices at the grocery store, at home, and when dining out requires some amount of open-mindedness and a willingness to develop new habits.

One key to healthier eating involves learning to cook—at least just a little. More satisfying, healthful eating can be easier if you learn how to prepare a few basic dishes that you enjoy and that can serve as stepping stones to more complex dishes. For example, learning how to sauté will open up your culinary repertoire to a huge range of quick and healthful vegetable, lean meat, and lower-fat dishes.

Cooking, beyond providing a healthier (and generally less costly) way to eat, can also be a gratifying activity. Cooking can also provide a way to enrich family life or to grow your social engagement. In addition to its health and gastronomic benefits, learning to cook a few basic dishes can also aid in weight control, if merely by limiting the amount and types of foods eaten away from home.

Americans today eat or drink more than a third of their total daily calories away from home. Such foods, whether prepared at take-out counters, fast-food emporiums, or tablecloth restaurants, tend to have higher amounts of salt, unhealthy fats, sugar, and calories than foods that are prepared and eaten at home.

Viewing food as medicine is not a new idea. Galen, a second-century Greek physician who became the most prominent and influential doctor in ancient Rome, maintained that good doctors should also be good cooks. Galen, who wrote *On the Power of Foods*, practiced and taught other healers to share recipes with their patients for their health. Integrative practitioners are often open to sharing recipes and dietary tips with their patients, a practice that is slowly gaining acceptance among mainstream providers as well.

Learning to cook a few basic dishes also helps keep you in charge of what you put into your body. If you're not the person in charge of cooking in your household, consider what you might do to support the person who does the cooking. For example, get involved with shopping smarter for the cook in your home, or become more involved as a menu planner or kitchen assistant (yes, cleanup counts too).

Many people who get into the kitchen—and especially those whose main job is to help devour new dishes—find it a wholesome and satisfying experience. Depending on your own or your household's nutritional needs, find books, videos, and instructional blogs online that can help you learn what you need to know to help make you a more relaxed, more skillful, and healthier cook.

Eating Right

Eating right is a common refrain—but what does that mean? Although the answer depends on your individual age, condition, health goals, budget, state of residence, preferences, and many other factors, a few basic truths apply to most people without significant food allergies, sensitivities, or diet-related health conditions:

Know the daily caloric intake recommended for your age, sex, and activity level.

New food and menu labels use 2,000 calories a day as a reference. However, your individual needs can vary, often quite significantly, especially if you are sedentary, middle-aged or older, or attempting to lose or gain weight. Use one of the many available calorie calculators to determine the approximate number of calories, on average, you should consume daily to maintain your weight at the same fitness level. Explore *http://fnic.nal.usda.gov* to learn more.

Keep an honest food and activity diary.

Use pen and paper, an app, or another electronic tool to record your entire food and drink intake over the course of a typical week, with emphasis on *typical*. Include everything that crosses your lips in truthful quantities, including alcoholic beverages and grazing snacks. Free apps such as MyFitnessPal that can track your net calories taken in (energy intake) and calories burned (energy expenditure) can help you identify where you may need to make modifications or improvements. Doing your own food and activity diary can be an enlightening, and perhaps sobering, experience. Wearable devices can help you track your activity level and may motivate you to walk more or burn more calories, too.

Fill up on fruits and vegetables.

Newer U.S. Department of Agriculture guidelines call for Americans to reconsider their breakfast, lunch, and dinner plates. Half of the meal should consist of fruits and vegetables, with the remainder made up of protein (preferably lean), grains (preferably whole grains), and a small amount of dairy products (preferably low fat and lower in sugar). A diet rich in raw, nutrient-rich, or healthfully cooked fruits and vegetables packs antioxidant, multivitamin, and nutrient power. If you can't remember many of the superfoods listed below, simply remember to shop and eat by color—the darker or more vivid the color of a fruit or vegetable, the generally higher its antioxidant and phytonutrient content is. Better yet, replace low-quality, high-calorie snacks or other junk foods that are low in nutritional value and loaded with added sugars with some of your favorite foods from the list below.

Adapt more healthful cooking methods.

Choose sautéing, roasting, pressure-cooking, and air-frying methods over deep-frying and other methods that leave your food soaked in large amounts of saturated animal or tropical fats. Swap out butter for olive oil and other plant oils with a healthier profile such as canola, grapeseed, nut, or safflower oils. Experiment with simple cooking methods that deliver big flavor and satisfying texture, such as poaching for fish and braising or roasting for meats. If you are short on time or live at a higher altitude or where energy costs are high, consider a modern, safety-enhanced pressure cooker, which conserves both nutrients and time.

Eat a diverse diet.

As creatures of habit, it's easy to slip into an eating rut. Such habits can result from or lead to boredom with a potential rebellious consequence: binge eating or indulging in poor eating choices. Consider having a meatless protein dish at least once a week as your main course—discover how delicious and protein-rich foods such as beans, nuts, soy, seitan, and higher protein grains such as farro and quinoa can be. Even eggs can be used creatively to substitute for meats, as in a baked vegetable-rich frittata. Ask your neighborhood green grocer about ways to prepare or serve different fruits or vegetables that are unfamiliar to you. With vegetables, simple roasting often does the trick, unlocking flavors that even veggie haters can love.

Experiment with herbs and spices.

Learn to build flavor with herbs and spices, including some you may not have tried before. Try something new every couple of weeks with a new herb or spice that can kick up food's flavors in unexpected ways. Combinations of cumin with cinnamon and paprika do wonders for ho-hum meat dishes, marinades, and stews. Or, blend herbs such as thyme leaves with olive oil, salt, and pepper and toss with winter vegetables such as cauliflower, squash, or carrots to make an easy, no-fuss oven-roasted dish that brings out their natural veggie sweetness along with savory highlights. Even if you don't consider yourself a creative cook, you can learn to boost flavor simply by using salt and pepper.

Choose real over processed foods.

Not only are real foods tasty and low in additives and chemicals, but they are also packed with many other nutrients your body needs besides vitamins and minerals. Such nutrients include the different types of fiber, essential fatty acids, micronutrients, fluids, antioxidants, phytochemicals, and flavonoids, which are typically found in a variety of fruits and vegetables as well as in tea and wine. This tip is especially important for people who need to curb their sodium intake. According to the CDC, the majority of American adults fall into this group, which includes all adults age 51 and older; all African Americans; and anyone with high blood pressure, chronic kidney disease, or any type of diabetes. A whopping 75% of Americans' salt intake comes from processed, prepackaged, and restaurant foods.

Choose nutrient-dense foods regularly.

Foods that are super-charged with a variety of nutrients and foods that supply hefty amounts of nutrients associated with a range of healthy effects are sometimes called superfoods. Whatever you choose to call them—how about delicious?—these nutrient-packed foods deserve a daily presence at mealtime. Consult your favorite food and recipe reference to find creative ways to bring these foods to your table.

Set your table with these examples of nutritious foods for health

Fruits
Apples
Avocados
Bananas/plantains
Berries (açai, blueberries, goji, raspberries, strawberries, others)
Cherries
Citrus
Grapes
Kiwi
Melons
Papaya
Pineapple
Pears

Vegetables
Bell peppers
Beets
Broccoli
Brussel sprouts
Dark greens (arugula, chard, collards, dandelion, kale, mustard, purslane, spinach)
Garlic, onions, shallots, chives, and leeks
Herbs (basil, rosemary, parsley, sage, thyme, marjoram, oregano, dill, bay leaf)
Hummus (tahini and garbanzo bean spread)
Mushrooms (portobello, crimini, and shiitake)
Potatoes (white or sweet)
Root vegetables (fennel, radish, celery root, salsify, carrots, parsnips, yams, turnips, kohlrabi)
Soybeans, other beans, lentils, and peas
Tofu

Eggs and Dairy
Cheese (ricotta, cottage, sheep and goat milk cheeses)
Eggs
Low-fat milk, kefir
Unsweetened or low-sugar yogurts (including Greek-style)

Grains, Seeds, and Nuts
Whole grains (barley, buckwheat, farro, bulgur, oats, quinoa, corn, rice, wheat)
Seeds (sesame, flax, chia, sunflower, hemp, pumpkin/pepitas)
Nuts (almonds, cashews, peanuts, walnuts, and others—preferably unsalted)

Meats
Fish, including fatty fish weekly (anchovies, salmon, black cod, sardines, canned light tuna, herring, trout, and less fatty fish such as shellfish, halibut, and various white flaky fishes)
Leaner cuts or types of meat (bison, flank, filet, pork tenderloin)
Poultry, preferably skinless and sustainably or organically raised

Other Foods, Condiments, and Spices
Chocolate, cacao, cocoa (less sweet or less processed versions)
Coffee and tea
Oils (olive, avocado, walnut, canola, grapeseed)
Seaweed (nori and others)
Spices (cinnamon, ginger, togarashi, turmeric, coriander, nutmeg, paprika, others)
Vitamin B-12–fortified nutritional yeast (especially for vegans)
Wheat germ

Eat mindfully.

This last tip is especially important for people who struggle with weight or whose eating behaviors set them up to fall into sugary, calorie-laden, high-fat food traps. Mindful eating is just that—being aware of the pleasure and nourishment of food in the moment. When applying mindfulness to eating, make yourself aware and appreciative of your nourishment by slowing down your eating, inviting savoring rather than scarfing. Open yourself up to noting the aromas, visual delights, contrasts, textures, flavors, and layers of your meal. Eat with purpose, and apply such mindfulness to your surroundings and to those at your table. Doing so will elevate eating to a shared and satisfying experience. An added benefit is that mindful eating has been shown to help with weight loss and maintenance.

WEIGHT CONTROL

A variety of alternative methods have been touted as weight control aids. Whether for losing weight or for building bulk, a steady stream of supplements cycle through the over-the-counter marketplace, promising *guaranteed, fat-burning, instant, incredible, dramatic, never-before* results, according to their marketing plugs. For the overwhelming majority of these weight control "cures," the evidence to support such claims is nonexistent. Moreover, many of these supplements have been found to contain either illegal prescription drugs, adulterants, stimulants, hormones, or possibly harmful herbal or chemical compounds. A significant number of FDA enforcement actions and recalls have involved such products, some of which (ephedra and others) have caused numerous deaths and serious side effects requiring hospitalization.

So which diet or weight control method works? Despite the revolving door of diet fads and the diet evangelists who maintain that their chosen dietary method is superior to others, the diet that works is the one that you can stick to. Ideally, that diet should be focused on real foods (and not food substitutes or heavily manipulated food-like substances) that are limited in added sugars, simple carbohydrates, saturated animal fats, excessive salt, and total calories. A sustainable and healthful weight-loss plan should offer a variety of foods that you enjoy; provide nutritional balance and include lean sources of protein, complex carbohydrates (which also promote a feeling of fullness or satiety), and nutrient-rich foods that are lower in calories or that can be enjoyed in smaller amounts (or both).

A Mediterranean-style diet has been associated with healthier living and health outcomes in multiple studies from study groups around the world. Typically, a Mediterranean diet includes ample fruits and vegetables, small amounts of lean meat, frequent servings of fish (at least twice weekly), healthy fats such as olive or canola oil, nuts, complex carbohydrates and grains, modest wine consumption, and the generous use of herbs and spices over the heavy use of salt or sugar.

Mediterranean nourishment generally translates into meals served at a table alongside other engaged people or family, often with some wine to share slowly and in moderation. Grazing, mindless eating, snacking, and eating in your car are not typical components of a Mediterranean diet. By applying creativity and personal preference to the use of herbs and spices, a Mediterranean-style diet can be adapted to reflect different ethnic preferences, from Nuevo Latino to Asian.

Can you match these decades to the diet fads of their day?

(Some fads were popular in more than one decade.)

Decade of popularity	Diet name or description
A. 1800s	1. Smoking diet
B. 19th century, early 1900s	2. Prayer diet
C. 1930s	3. Grapefruit diet
D. 1940s	4. Tapeworm diet
E. 1950s	5. Low-fat diets
F. 1960s	6. Master cleansing diets
G. 1970s	7. Cabbage soup diet
H. 1980s	8. Eating by blood type
I. 1990s	9. Diet pills
J. 2000s	10. Low-carb, high protein diets
K. 2010s	11. Vinegar diet
	12. Food-combining diets
	13. Chewing diets (Fletcherism)
	14. HCG diet
	15. Diet potions
	16. Anti-inflammatory diet
	17. No-grain or gluten-free diets
	18. Drinking man's diet
	19. Zone, Atkins, and South Beach diets
	20. Low-calorie diets
	21. Weight loss clubs, support groups

Answers: A. 4, 9, 11, 15; B. 4, 13, 15; C. 1; D. 6; E. 2, 3; F. 7, 18, 21; G. 6, 9, 20; H. 5; I. 8, 10; J. 6, 19; K. 14, 16, 17.

Work with your health-care provider or a registered dietician to find a plan that works for you. Ideally, such a plan will consider your specific health status and weight loss or weight gain goals. Consider also your activity level, lifestyle, food triggers or traps, and family and employment situation, along with other factors that can influence your commitment, your adaptability to change, and the sustainability of that diet plan.

Despite decades of claims to the contrary, a safe and effective weight loss aid has yet to emerge from either the pharmaceutical or the nutraceutical realm. Instead of looking toward injectable or oral solutions for weight control, whose safety and effectiveness are iffy at best and risky at worst, choose to make meaningful lifestyle and behavioral adjustments that are durable, are healthful, and bring long-term rewards beyond the cosmetic.

Eating high-fiber foods—in combination with other healthy foods—appears to aid in weight loss, and is safe for most people without digestive problems. Increasing the amount of fiber-rich foods in the diet helps you feel fuller. Fiber also helps slow down overeating or mindless eating when you are no longer hungry. Soluble fibers, typically found in foods such as beans, tree fruits, and nuts, can also help lower cholesterol, especially the "bad" LDL (low-density lipoprotein) cholesterol. If you are among the vast majority of Americans who do not obtain the recommended 21 to 38 grams of fiber in their daily diets, consider supplementing your diet with ground flaxseed or psyllium. Both are readily available over the counter in forms that may be used with liquids or for use on or in other foods.

A few integrative methods appear promising for weight control. However, these methods may have higher success rates when they are woven into a nutritional or behavioral care plan that includes portion control, physical activity, nutritional counseling, and healthful dietary modifications. Learn more about these specific methods in other sections of this book and in the "Where to Learn More" references.

Alternative Approaches to Weight Loss

Yoga*
Mindfulness*
Hypnosis**
Relaxation therapies**
Ayurveda
Acupuncture
Chinese medicine

*Methods associated with relatively stronger evidence.
**Methods that may be useful as part of an integrative approach to cravings, binging, and eating disorders.

Although a variety of nutritional supplements and products have been touted in the media, at gyms, and by different types of nutritionists (who may or may not have been formally trained in nutrition science) as alternative methods of weight loss, evidence of their effectiveness is scant. Such products whose weight loss claims still remain to be proven include açai berry, green coffee bean extract, human chorionic gonadotropin (HCG), and raspberry ketones, among others. A few studies have shown weight loss associated with green tea, both as a beverage and as a purified extract; however, the weight loss was minor and may not be significant in a long-term or real-life setting.

Sleep: A Vital Sign?

An overlooked contributor to weight control and other overall health problems is sleep, specifically inadequate or poor-quality sleep. Too little sleep has been associated with obesity in children as well as adults. For overall health and to aid in successful weight management, strive to adopt regular sleep habits. Aim for about seven to eight hours of sleep nightly (more in young children and teenagers).

Other tips for better sleep include eating dinner at least two, and preferably three or more, hours before bedtime. Create an environment that promotes uninterrupted, comfortable, and restful sleep sheltered from noise, distraction, and light. Limit intense visual stimulation before bedtime, such as television viewing, emailing/texting, playing video games, and other types of screen time. Consider adopting a ritual that allows you to wind down before bedtime, too, whether it's reading, listening to calming music, meditating, or using another relaxation strategy that helps you decompress and let go of the day.

Catch Your ZZZs

Below is a partial list of factors or conditions that are aggravated or influenced by a lack of sleep or poor sleep quality. Be diligent about sticking to a regular sleep schedule for your overall health and safety and to promote healthier aging.

Accidents and errors	Immune function
Alzheimer's disease onset and progression	Inflammation
	Insulin sensitivity
Behavior, emotions, and mood	Learning, mental clarity
Blood pressure	Mortality
Breathing disorders	Obesity
Depression	Risky behaviors
Diabetes	Smoking
Heart disease; heart disease and stroke risk	

EXERCISE

Our 21st-century sedentary lifestyles are taking an enormous toll on our health. Globally, physical inactivity is a major risk to public health as well as individual and economic prosperity. The lack of adequate physical activity increases the risk for a range of chronic diseases and conditions such as heart disease and stroke, diabetes, obesity, osteoporosis, high blood pressure, and certain forms of cancer involving the colon and breast. Balance and the risk of falls are also affected by more sitting and less movement.

Prolonged television viewing and screen time in front of computers and other electronic devices are associated with higher weight (as measured by body mass index, or BMI), lower fitness levels, higher blood cholesterol, and even an increased risk for premature death.

Individuals who care about their health and seize the opportunity to make improvements to their level of fitness stand to reap great benefits to their overall physical and mental health from greater physical activity.

Fortunately, recent studies have shown that people who engage in short bursts of intense exercise can also reap the health benefits of exercise. These seven- or 14-minute workouts, as they are popularly known, can be suitable for individuals who have limited time for exercise or for people who travel frequently. Such activity contributes to the aerobic fitness of the heart and lung systems, muscle strength, and balance. Discuss these options with your health-care provider before embarking on more intense forms of exercise, especially if you have heart problems or risk factors, if you have orthopedic problems, or if you are not used to exercising.

For those who choose to participate in more traditional forms of activity, such as biking, swimming, running, tennis, and the like, the World Health Organization guidelines call for 30 minutes of moderate activity at least five times per week, in addition to your usual activities.

Some forms of physical activity are also ripe opportunities to initiate or boost social connectivity, which is associated with greater levels of happiness and lower levels of depression and withdrawal. Being involved in an exercise or activity group such as formal or informal biking, hiking, or walking clubs also contributes to group safety and can support successful aging.

Disabled persons or those with limited mobility may be especially interested in alternative forms of physical activity. These can include chair yoga, water therapy (hydrotherapy), and the slow-movement Chinese practice of tai chi.

HEALTHY HABITS/LIFESTYLE

Habits are tough to break, and new ones can be even tougher to form. However, opening our eyes to the precious gift of health can guide the way toward better living. Strive to rid yourself of habits and environments that are not positive or life enhancing. If you struggle with weight, consider limiting time with acquaintances who tend to overeat, a factor that has been associated with further weight gain. Even without making big or rapid changes, strive to develop better habits that foster better physical and mental health, perhaps day by day or a small step at a time.

Consider taking a fresh look at certain outlooks and attitudes that have been associated with greater levels of happiness, serenity, and successful aging. These include the following:

Gratitude

Feeling truly grateful for what we have has been tied to greater serenity, mindfulness, well-being, and overall happiness. Feeling and expressing thankfulness also helps us to develop stronger and more meaningful relationships, both personally and at work. Having a sense of gratitude can also help us to manage stress better. Cultivate an attitude of gratitude, even through difficult times, whether through prayer, meditation, professional guidance, or your own method.

Optimism

Between personal difficulties, life's uncertainties, and global tumult, feeling optimistic can be challenging. Strive to avoid negative thoughts and beliefs and to find the good in daily life to reaffirm your sense of optimism through tough times. Meditation and mind-body practices can help in opening yourself up to greater optimism.

Connectivity

Even for loners, a sense of connection is an important element of the human condition. Look to make that connection by engaging with other people, loved ones, pets, and causes. Social engagement can be energizing and life enhancing and can also help stave off depression and negativism. Friends and acquaintances can help you weave more or new types of physical, spiritual, or intellectual activities into your daily life and ramp up the fun in such undertakings.

Passion

Having a passion and indulging that passion can be profoundly satisfying, energizing, and life affirming. Set time aside from your busy home or work life to develop, identify, or feed your passion, whether through the arts, sports, cooking, or other avenues of personal expression.

Spirituality

Often related to connectivity, spirituality is highly individual. Regardless of religious affiliation, many people find spiritual satisfaction through yoga, meditation, prayer walking, some mind-body practices, and whole systems of care such as Chinese medicine and Ayurveda.

Acceptance

A great deal of mental energy in the early part of our lives is spent deciphering the whys of the world. As we move into middle age and beyond, the answers to the whys of life can appear fuzzier, or perhaps unanswerable. Judicious acceptance can help smooth out some of life's rough edges, and help us deal with the inevitability of change.

Switch Off to Detoxify

Finally, although specific detoxifying methods are discussed in Chapter 11, another type of detoxification is also important to healthier living. This type of detoxification involves freeing yourself from an obsession with famous people, media culture, and the daily diet of noxious stimuli presented to us on-screen and through other media, whether print or electronic. Detox from dark dramas with unkind themes and from so-called entertainment that is focused on violent acts, negativity, or unsavory aspects of human behavior.

A 2014 study by the Nielsen media conglomerate found that the average American spends five hours per day watching television. With aging, that number climbs to seven hours daily for seniors, not counting other electronic activities involving smartphones, computers, and radio.

Instead, consider choosing to spend your precious leisure time more fruitfully by indulging in and supporting nonviolent, kinder, and more life-affirming entertainment. Find diversion in learning something new or finding more ways to enhance your health through giving, personal development, positive messaging, love, and support for others.

WHERE TO LEARN MORE

Handy and easy-to-use references to determine your caloric needs, dietary reference intakes for nutrients, body-mass index, and more: *http://fnic.nal.usda.gov*

A visual way to help you eat healthier, plus resources on dieting, smart shopping, recipes, tips, and tracking tools to keep you on a healthier eating path: *http://www.choosemyplate.gov*

Fun, free, and informative resources courtesy of Brian Wansink, Ph.D., an expert and creative change agent on eating behaviors: *http://mindlesseating.org*

Life's Simple 7, an action plan for healthier living and heart health from the American Heart Association: *http://mylifecheck.heart.org*

Physical activity guidelines and tips, including yoga and other practices: *http://www.health.gov/paguidelines/*

Tips, articles, videos, and more about gratitude and cultivating a more meaningful life: *http://greatergood.berkeley.edu*

Dietary Guidelines for the Brazilian Population, 2014, which has been cited as one of the world's most intelligent food guides, regardless of ethnicity: *http://189.28.128.100/dab/docs/portaldab/publicacoes/guia_alimentar_populacao_ingles.pdf*

United Kingdom National Institute for Health and Care Excellence: *www.nice.org.uk/*

Social Determinants of Health 2008, World Health Organization: *www.who.int/social_determinants/thecommission/finalreport/en/*

13

Myths and Misconceptions

THROUGHOUT THIS BOOK, WE'VE EXPLORED MANY MISCONCEPTIONS AND myths about what works and what does not. Here, we explore a few myths that you may have heard, believed, or wondered about regarding alternative, integrative, and mainstream medical care.

Although this chapter has been divided into myths regarding alternative and integrative approaches and those with respect to conventional Western medicine, certain aspects of these myths could be relevant to both areas.

Understanding that we tend to remember facts that reinforce our basic beliefs—and forget or not register facts that are not in sync with our belief system or way of thinking—here are a few myths that may challenge you to consider matters in a different way.

MYTHS ABOUT INTEGRATIVE AND ALTERNATIVE MEDICINE

Myth: Natural products are better for you.

Intuitively, it seems correct that a natural product will be better for you than an artificial or man-made substitute. It's also easy for a product, food, or service to claim it is natural because that word has no legally binding meaning. But, as many examples from nature show us—whether it's poison hemlock, mercury, or ultraviolet rays from sunshine—just because something exists in nature or is natural does not automatically make it nontoxic or better for you.

This is a hard myth to dispel, even though it contains an ounce of truth. While it is surely preferable to choose a remedy that is gentler, less invasive, and as nontoxic as possible while still being effective, many natural remedies are none of the above. This can be especially true with dietary supplements that are adulterated or spiked with prescription drugs or made in a way that allows the finished product that you ingest to contain toxic substances such as lead or other heavy metals from the plant's environment. Chapter 9 explains other safety and ethical concerns with supplements.

You could also challenge yourself to consider whether a natural therapy of any kind that you use instead of a therapy that has been proven to work safely is truly a nontoxic or suitable choice.

For example, is it wise for a cancer patient who has the choice of a conventional therapy with a good potential for cure or extending their survival to miss a critical window of treatment opportunity to pursue a therapy considered to be more natural, and possibly of questionable benefit?

These are difficult questions, and it can be challenging to uncover the best answer. Bring up your concerns with your health-care team. You might be surprised about how much they know about many natural remedies or how interested they are to hear out your concerns and preferences. Ask them to work together with you to arrive at a truly integrated care plan.

Myth: If an alternative practice has not been shown to be effective, even if it is safe and low-cost, don't use it.

Population studies that provide or fail to show the evidence upon which recommendations are based are just that: studies done on populations. Headlines often proclaim that a remedy is effective or not effective without taking into consideration how many people were studied—10 or 10,000—or whether the design of the study itself was flawed. Recommendations that are based on evidence take these numbers and other factors into account.

Many studies are observational, meaning that a certain population was studied over time and the data were teased out from their habits, behaviors, and associated health conditions. In contrast, a controlled clinical trial takes different groups and tests them against groups that don't receive the treatment and/or groups that receive a placebo treatment.

Another type of study relates to comparisons—that is, how effective one treatment may be in comparison to another. An example might be acupuncture versus yoga for fibromyalgia, instead of testing acupuncture against a prescription drug in a randomized, controlled trial with a placebo.

Our understanding of what works and to what degree with respect to alternative medicine and integrative practices remains fairly basic. Many more studies are needed in larger and different groups of people before results can be better generalized to the population at large, beyond those of scientific or observational studies.

Although in general it doesn't make much sense to pursue therapies that have not been shown to be effective, it's also important to remember that usually, such therapies have not been shown to be effective in most people, most of the time, over the course of a study or in many studies. Yet in reality, some individuals may benefit from a therapy that hasn't worked for others, as we see with conventional drugs and practices all the time. Health-care professionals treat the individual patient sitting before them, and that person might be the outlier who might indeed respond to the therapy that did not work for most of the people in a treatment group of a trial.

Recall that a wise choice of any treatment method should always consider those that hit the sweet spot of safety, effectiveness, and tolerability. Also important is adherence—that is, how well you will be able to embark on and stick to the recommended therapy. After all, if you are unable to follow a treatment or diet as suggested, no matter how well it's been proven to work in others, the chances of it working for you are pretty slim.

Consider safety first when considering alternative treatments that have not been shown to be effective or that have questionable efficacy, especially with regard to their safety in people like you. For example, if you are diabetic and are considering an alternative treatment that hasn't been shown to work well but that you are eager to try in order to avoid using insulin, stay away from treatments or supplements that have been shown to be risky when used by diabetics, such as yohimbe.

Also, consider the cost and how committed you believe you can be to that method. If you are not likely to follow through on the regimen, it may not make sense to take on the risk associated with that therapy, especially without allowing yourself the chance to reap the full benefit, if any.

Be sure to discuss unproven, new, and potentially helpful therapies that you are considering with your health-care team. Bring any research you've uncovered with you, and help your team understand why you want to pursue the option and what you consider the risks and benefits to be.

Myth: I can do my own research and determine risks and benefits independently.

While that belief may be true at face value, studies show that much of the information we glean from common sources such as the Internet, health-focused publications, and medical television is inaccurate.

A 2014 Canadian study of medical television found that evidence that was believable or somewhat believable only existed for about one out of three or at most one out of two recommendations. That's a coin toss. Evidence was nonexistent for the recommendations given about 25–33% of the time. Even less frequent were the comments made during the program about the amount of benefit that might be expected of the specific treatments or supplements. Less often still was any mention of side effects, potential conflicts of interest, and cost issues.

Given that the average show in the study doled out 11 to 12 recommendations per episode, such a high level of inaccurate, potentially conflicted and incomplete information is concerning. TV doctors have been dressed down before Congress for overstating the benefits of supplements and certain therapies, and for mistaking unfounded claims for proven effectiveness. At least one TV doctor has drawn the ire, and multiple warning letters, from the FDA for making illegal claims about his products.

A separate study about information for high blood pressure found that about one-third of videos on YouTube gave inaccurate information, including that related to a host of dietary supplements, nutritionals (notably L-arginine), massage, and acupuncture.

In another study of common herbal products that reviewed nearly 1,200 websites, researchers found that safety information, including possible side effects and interactions with drugs, was provided by less than 8% of the sites. Only 3% of the websites provided scientific references to back up their claims, and only one in 10 suggested consultation with a health-care practitioner.

Another factor standing in the way of objectively assessing health information that is available through the media is the fact that many people already have preconceived notions. Such beliefs, whether they pertain to mainstream or other forms of medicine, may color their interpretation of health issues and news.

For example, a recent study found that nearly one in four U.S. adults believe that, as stated in the survey question, the FDA is withholding natural cures for cancer from the American public because it is under the thumb of large drug companies. Another 10–20% of respondents believed there were other secret or conspiracy agendas behind vaccination policies, water fluoridation, and the food supply. When such beliefs are tightly held, it can be difficult to reconcile facts and the truth.

Regarding risks and benefits, a late 2014 study showed that health consumers tended to overestimate the benefits of standard medical treatments and to underestimate the potential harmful consequences of therapies. Understanding that consumers received such information from doctors who had described possible risks and harms, it is likely that self-directed health consumers who are considering alternative or unproven therapies on their own may be interpreting information through the filter of their own biases or beliefs, overestimating benefits and underestimating risks even more.

Finally, health care involves many complex decisions, many of which befuddle even the smartest, most up-to-date, and most highly trained professionals. Not only does a comprehensive understanding demand a high level of scientific literacy, but it also demands diverse experiences with many different types of patients and well-trained colleagues, a solid understanding of statistics and probabilities, and an appreciation for the limitations of research and data.

Notwithstanding all the biases and difficulties, it is wise to pursue your own research. Become as well informed as you can about your health and health options. Then, take it a step further by establishing communication with your health-care team to explore and resolve your concerns, what you've learned, and how you want to proceed along an integrative path.

Myth: Diplomas prove that providers are trained and certified.

You've probably seen the walls of a health-care practitioner's office covered in diplomas, certificates, and perhaps awards. What do they mean, if anything?

One way to find out would be to ask the practitioner, although that's hardly the best use of your scheduled time. Ahead of your visit, however, you can do some exploring to find out where or whether your providers trained, the range of their experience, and what kind of license or certification they hold.

This can be a frustrating area for health consumers to decipher because the respectability and professionalism of many diploma-granting societies can vary widely. Diploma mills are common. Online testimonials are often scripted, unreliable, purchased, or irrelevant to your care. Providers may be self-taught or have had little or limited structured training. Some providers may not have been tested or evaluated for their basic fund of knowledge or competence, or perhaps have not passed the corresponding examinations in their field of practice.

Some societies with impressive-sounding names require little more than the payment of a fee. Certain "best" and "top doctor" awards and citations are given out if the individual applies and pays the fee—much like advertising.

This situation can also pertain to mainstream medical doctors and practitioners. Although they may be board-certified by an established board that is recognized by the American Board of Medical Specialties (ABMS), they may also have received training or certification by organizations or boards that are not, not yet, or perhaps never will be recognized by the ABMS.

Such ABMS recognition may not be that important if, for example, you seek a practitioner who is qualified in biofeedback or another specialized therapy. In such cases, determine what the practitioners' baseline qualifications are in treating patients like you, and whether they have been adequately trained and certified by a respected, ethical association or organization recognized for excellence in that field.

Use the references to established associations and organizations throughout the book to learn more about your practitioner's licensing, certification, and training.

MYTHS ABOUT CONVENTIONAL WESTERN MEDICINE

Myth: Alternative practices don't really work—and when they seem to work, it's just a placebo effect.

As many sections of this book have already shown, an array of alternative and integrative practices do indeed have beneficial effects that are meaningful compared to the benefits obtained through mainstream practices. Further, many therapies not considered mainstream can enhance conventional care, providing even greater benefit to the patient. What's more, many of these benefits often come at lower cost and with a greater safety margin because of lower toxicity and a lower risk of side effects. That's what integrative care is all about.

Among the many examples examined in this book are massage, acupuncture, and chiropractic for lower back pain, as well as a variety of mind-body techniques for anxiety, pain, and even blood pressure control.

Honing in on whether the benefits merely signify placebo effects, it's important to appreciate that mainstream practitioners are beginning to take a closer and appreciative look at placebos. After all, the benefits from placebos are not trifling, reaching 50% or more in some studies. Recent research has shown that placebos do indeed excite important centers of the brain that are related to the release of endorphins. Besides, sham treatments using placebos do not have a neutral effect on the brain. Rather, placebos have been shown to trigger brain and body signaling that, although different from the pathways turned on by the genuine treatment being studied, was nevertheless important and might help to explain why some people appear to respond to a placebo treatment.

A curious 2007 study on the power of placebos, in this case merely a suggestion, was done with 84 hotel room attendants. After only four weeks, the group that had been informed that the cleaning work that they were doing was good exercise, and that it met the active lifestyle recommendations of the Surgeon General, reported that they felt as though they were getting much more exercise than before. Moreover, the counseled group weighed less and had lower blood pressure, body fat, and body mass indexes compared to the group that had not received such counseling.

Another important factor in healing of any kind is whether or not the person being treated is engaged or actively participating in the treatment plan and whether they feel encouraged, validated, and supported by their provider. Many integrative practitioners take the time to develop interpersonal relationships and have more open communication with their patients about many different aspects of their health. Using warmth, interest, and even simple touch, such providers aim to establish an emotional bond with their patients.

Connection and communication have been shown to help individuals feel more involved with their care. With involvement comes a type of shared ownership, in contrast to the paternalistic, passive, or more controlling methods often encountered in mainstream medicine. Warmer, more personal integrative care models tend to produce better results with many different types of chronic conditions, from pain syndromes to depression. Whether this occurs because patients feel and act more responsibly about sticking to the treatment plan or whether the positive outcomes may relate in part to the placebo response have not been fully explained.

Myth: The U.S. has the best health-care system in the world.

In terms of technology, that might be true. However, in terms of results, the statement above is indeed a myth. If you compare statistics of how the U.S. fares in measurements such as infant **mortality**, longevity, and death rates from a variety of conditions—for which mainstream medicine possesses a vast and often high-tech armamentarium—versus countries that are considered our peers such as Japan, the United Kingdom, Australia, Israel, and other nations, we fall very short of being number one, except in spending and obesity.

A study from the Organization for Economic Cooperation and Development reporting on its 34 members in 2012 showed that the U.S. ranked second in diabetes prevalence, seventh in cancer incidence, ninth in preventing death from cancer, 25th in preventing death from heart disease, 27th in life expectancy, 31st in infant mortality, and 31st in preventing premature death.

Among a smaller group of nine nations from North America, Europe, and Oceania, the U.S. was third in the average length of time spent waiting to see a specialist, trailing behind Germany and Switzerland.

Despite leading this group of advanced nations in spending (and nearly leading in waiting time), our health-care system does not deliver what payers of top dollar should expect, especially with regard to chronic diseases. We can and must do better.

Myth: If you ask for a second opinion regarding integrative care, your doctor will get mad at you.

Perhaps that's not entirely a myth, since that has and could happen. However, as mainstream medical care evolves toward more inclusive and cooperative practices that entertain a wider range of therapies from a variety of fields to foster better outcomes for patients, chances are improving that this will occur less often.

Second opinions are underused in medicine in many different scenarios and for many reasons. Often, patients may wish to avoid the risk of offending a doctor with whom they may have a bond or whom they wish to continue seeing, regardless of the outcome of the second opinion.

Doctors are more accustomed to requests for second opinions when it comes to major surgery, cancer, or difficult diagnoses. Increasingly, patients are asking for second opinions regarding integrative care, notably for integrative oncology care. Many medical centers have brought integrative oncology care onboard or are at least familiar with it.

Like any other type of health-care professional, mainstream physicians want their patients to be happy, to feel comfortable, and to understand their care. They want their patients to experience the best possible outcome at the least possible risk—and they also want their patients to feel comfortable and secure in their care.

When approaching the question of a second opinion with your doctor, keep these factors in mind and express them as a collaborator or partner in your care. Do your homework ahead of time so that you are able to state the methods that appeal to you or present a few options or providers that interest you. Ask your physician for help in creating an integrative plan for your health. Most reasonable physicians will be understanding and should appreciate and respect your interest in taking a greater, more involved role in your care.

Myth: If you take a prescription drug and it doesn't work, try something else.

It's been estimated that half of all patients do not take their medications as prescribed or not at all. What's more, half or more of all prescriptions written are not filled by the pharmacy, and up to about 20% of all prescriptions are not even picked up. The bottom line is that only about one in five people may be getting the intended benefit from prescription drugs—a considerable waste of health-care efforts and expenditures.

What's worse, perhaps, is that people who do not take their medications as instructed risk going in the hospital for unwanted reactions known as adverse drug events. In one study, adverse drug events that resulted in a hospital admission were tied to poor medication compliance in nearly seven out of 10 cases.

The risks of being hospitalized, rehospitalized, or dying prematurely are also much higher in people who don't take their medicines as intended, compared to those who do. Taking high blood pressure as one example, these risks are a staggering five times higher in people who don't take their medicines as prescribed.

The reasons given for not taking medications as intended, called **nonadherence**, are many. Sometimes the instructions are too complicated or the patient did not fully understand how they were supposed to take his or her medicines. Patients who do not feel ill, as with those with some forms of high blood pressure, high cholesterol, or diabetes, may be less interested in taking their medicines, especially if they experience side effects from them or do not feel the benefit. For others, cost or inconvenience may be barriers affecting their medication adherence.

The human and financial costs of nonadherence are high, tagged to 125,000 deaths per year and an estimated nearly $300 billion in health-care costs.

Explain any issues you may be having regarding your medications and supplements to your health-care team, especially if you don't fully understand or accept the instructions given by your doctor. A physician assistant, pharmacist, or nurse practitioner may also be able to explain how to take your medications correctly or to help you and your provider find a suitable alternative.

Pharmacists possess a wealth of information about drugs, side effects, and alternatives. They also are well informed about interactions and the best way to take your medicines, especially if you are trying to juggle multiple dosing schedules. Consult them and keep good records about what you learn. They can offer tips to make adherence easier, or they may suggest a lower-cost option or a schedule that will make it easier for you to take your drugs and supplements the right way for the best possible result.

Myth: Mainstream medicine is mostly based on evidence and all other types of health practices are not, whether alternative or integrative.

Perhaps this is the biggest myth of all, assumed to be true by many health consumers as well as by many mainstream practitioners. The fact is that neither part of that sentence is correct—most mainstream medical practices actually fall into the gray zone of evidence, neither definitively proven nor totally debunked. Similarly, most of the other types of health practices explored in this book also fall into the gray zone, with some appearing more promising than others.

Many reasons exist for this situation. These include the difficulties in performing well-funded and cleanly designed studies over long periods of time in large groups of people who complete the entire study—and that are done with no conflicts of interest—yielding statistically sound data that delivers clear-cut and unambiguous results. Few studies are that ideal.

Another reason involves progress itself. As tests, procedures, or new medicines become more familiar to practitioners and health consumers, the demand for them tends to increase, leading practitioners to use the new treatments in new groups of people. These new populations may not have been the target or study group in whom they were originally tested and from where the evidence or approval derived. Once the use of a treatment expands to more types of people or to greater numbers of people, it may take many years to find out that a therapy that performed well in, for example, middle-aged people has no effect—or might even be harmful—when used in seniors, or that a new therapy works well in men but has only average or poor performance in women, as has been found with some types of cardiac care.

At other times, it is patients themselves who may choose a therapy that has not been shown to be as effective as standard care out of their own personal preference or beliefs. Physicians also may have their own preferences about certain surgical, testing, or treatment approaches that may not be well supported by evidence but are believed to work in that doctor's hands (or mind). Sometimes, maybe they do. And sometimes, evidence is in the eye of the beholder.

FINDING YOUR HEALING WAYS

As explored in these pages, there are many ways to further health and wellness. Even in the face of serious disease, options abound for care that is integrative, patient-centered, and responsive to your needs.

In deciding the best path for you, begin by opening up communication with your health-care provider or team. Become as well educated as you feel comfortable doing to better understand your health and to help point you toward more informed decisions. The more you understand your condition and your own body, the better equipped you may feel to weigh the different options available and to follow a plan of action.

Progress in our understanding of health, disease, and treatments continues to evolve, as do the levels of evidence for many therapies—whether mainstream or otherwise. Evidence is a work in progress. Although progress can come with greater complexity of care, as we are beginning to see with genetic testing, so much of good health and good care remains based on a few simple tenets regarding optimal healthy living and lifestyle choices. Attitude, feeling gratitude, being connected, and yes, even love are also powerful forces for health, happiness, and successful aging. Use all of these to grow and preserve your health.

Understand that as knowledge about health expands and as challenges to health increase, uncertainties will always exist. Wrong decisions are sometimes made, even in the public eye. Experts will argue back and forth about what the best or right way is until evidence has grown sufficiently to make the conclusion clear and acceptable—until it's changed again by new knowledge or experiences. The Ebola crisis was yet another reminder of how difficult it can be to cope with medical uncertainty when new health challenges emerge, especially in real time and squarely in the public eye. Surely there will be others.

Reconsider how you care for your body and nurture your soul on a regular basis. Ask yourself if you are doing all you can do to foster allover health and wellness. Be honest with yourself, or talk it over with a trusted friend or mentor. If it appears that you could be doing more, find a way to get on track to approach health differently and sustainably toward successful outcomes.

The goal for this book was to help readers understand and appreciate the power we have in maintaining and improving our health, whether by using the force of the mind-body connection, ancient healing remedies, the magic of touch, delectable and wholesome nutrition, or another method. Another goal was to inspire readers toward greater health in many aspects of life beyond doctor visits and products.

Many wise individuals who have experienced serious illness will tell you that without health, many things that seemed important tend to lose their primacy. Health becomes what matters, perhaps above all. Endeavor to not take your health for granted, possibly using a daily affirmation. By considering health as your most precious treasure, you can explore and pursue ways to provide your mind, body, and spirit with the attention, love, and nurturing it needs to sustain the whole of you as a vital force for years to come.

14

Integrative Method Finder

A S EVIDENCE ABOUT DIFFERENT INTEGRATIVE METHODS CONTINUES TO EMERGE and shift, use this method finder to begin looking into the healing ways that suit your needs. Because new studies are bound to emerge, a therapy that may not appear to work today may indeed look more promising tomorrow.

Consider this chart a work in progress; use it to add your own information and that of your health-care team.

Topics such as good nutrition, adequate sleep, physical activity, clean living, and a positive outlook that are discussed in Chapter 12 and elsewhere are not listed in the finder because all of these have the power to help just about any condition. Some of these choices may be more powerful as preventive measures, and others may help more with healing or coping. Use them to their maximum potential.

The listing that follows is selective and is not meant to be complete. Whole systems of care such as naturopathy and traditional Chinese medicine are not prominently featured here because these methods often employ a combination of specific therapies or herbs in the care of an individual. Consult the chapters on those topics to learn more.

Additional information about what appears to work or not work is found throughout the book. Consult the corresponding chapters to review more specific information about certain subtypes of conditions or methods that are included under the more general terms used in the finder headings.

As with all the information in this book, weigh what you learn carefully in the context of your individual situation. Inform your health-care team about your interests and preferences to find the optimal, safest paths to health.

INTEGRATIVE METHOD FINDER

Condition or Focus	Evidence*	Methods or supplements
Acne	Moderate	Tea tree oil
Allergy/sinusitis	Supportive	Butterbur
	Moderate	Acupuncture, bromelain
	Low	Homeopathy, osteopathic manipulation
Alzheimer's disease	Supportive	Music therapy
	Moderate	Ginseng, massage
	Low	Reflexology, curcumin, ginkgo
Anxiety	Supportive	Mind-body, yoga, meditation, biofeedback, massage, guided imagery, hypnosis
	Moderate	Melatonin, Reiki
	Low	St. John's wort, aromatherapy, Rolfing
Arthritis (osteoarthritis)	Supportive	Acupuncture, tai chi
	Moderate	Yoga, massage, electromagnetic therapy
	Low	Glucosamine/chondroitin, bromelain, ginger, fish oil
Arthritis (rheumatoid)	Supportive	Biofeedback, meditation, mind-body, yoga, tai chi
	Moderate	Ayurveda, traditional Chinese medicine, fish oil
Asthma (nonacute)	Supportive	———
	Moderate	Mind-body, acupuncture, guided imagery
	Low	Yoga, butterbur, fish oil
Blood pressure	Supportive	Mind-body, yoga, meditation, biofeedback, CoQ10, fish oil, tai chi
	Moderate	Magnesium, ginseng
	Low	Chiropractic, probiotics
Bone health	Supportive	Magnesium, vitamin D, calcium, tai chi
	Moderate	Fish oil
	Low	DHEA

Condition or Focus	Evidence*	Methods or supplements
Cancer care	Supportive	Mind-body, guided imagery, hypnotherapy, massage
	Moderate	Acupuncture, meditation, yoga, curcumin, green tea, glutamine, maitake mushrooms, fish oil, milk thistle, astragalus, melatonin, probiotics, vitamin D, massage
	Low	Ashwagandha, ginger, Reiki, reflexology
Chronic illness	Supportive	Guided imagery, mind-body
Colds	Moderate	Vitamin C (to decrease severity, duration)
	Low	Echinacea, probiotics, homeopathy
Constipation	Moderate	Biofeedback, massage
Depression	Supportive	Yoga, St. John's wort (mild to moderate depression), music therapy, mind-body, meditation, acupuncture
	Moderate	Tai chi, qi gong, Ayurveda, ginseng, massage, electromagnetic therapy
	Low	Aromatherapy, Feldenkrais, St. John's wort (major depression), fish oil (perinatal depression)
Diabetes or metabolic syndrome	Moderate	Cinnamon, magnesium, fish oil, acupuncture (for peripheral neuropathy), ginger, ginseng
	Low	Milk thistle, reflexology, ashwagandha
Diarrhea	Supportive	Probiotics
End-of-life care	Supportive	Guided imagery, gentle manual therapies
Fibromyalgia	Supportive	Yoga, acupuncture, massage, mind-body
	Moderate	Tai chi, guided imagery, qi gong, biofeedback, hypnosis, electromagnetic therapy
	Low	Homeopathy, dietary supplements, chiropractic, magnet therapy, Rolfing
Gastrointestinal health	Supportive	Nutrition therapy, fiber
	Moderate	Probiotics, curcumin
	Low	Chiropractic

Condition or Focus	Evidence*	Methods or supplements
Headache	Supportive	Butterbur (migraine), biofeedback, massage, acupuncture, tai chi, mind-body
	Moderate	Chiropractic spinal manipulation, guided imagery, osteopathic manipulation
	Low	Chiropractic (without manipulation), hypnotherapy
Heart health	Supportive	Mind-body, fish oil, meditation, tai chi
	Moderate	Magnesium, CoQ10
	Low	Probiotics, most nonvitamin, nonmineral supplements
Immune support	Moderate	Guided imagery, mind-body, tai chi
	Low	Probiotics, aromatherapy, DHEA (lupus)
Incontinence (fecal)	Moderate	Biofeedback
Inflammatory bowel disorders	Supportive	Probiotics (ulcerative colitis)
	Moderate	Mind-body, curcumin (ulcerative colitis)
	Low	Peppermint oil, acupuncture, homeopathy
Insomnia	Supportive	Yoga, mind-body, tai chi
	Moderate	Melatonin, electromagnetic therapy
	Low	Acupuncture, massage, chiropractic
Irritable bowel syndrome	Supportive	Probiotics, hypnotherapy, mind-body
	Moderate	Guided imagery, meditation, osteopathic manipulation
	Low	Peppermint oil, acupuncture, homeopathy
Liver	Moderate	Milk thistle, fish oil
Lower back pain	Supportive	Yoga, chiropractic spinal manipulation, acupuncture, massage, osteopathic manipulation
	Moderate	Alexander technique
Memory	Low	Ginkgo

Condition or Focus	Evidence*	Methods or supplements
Menopausal symptoms	Supportive	Mind-body
	Moderate	Yoga, black cohosh, St. John's wort, ginseng, meditation, hypnotherapy
Menstrual pain/PMS	Supportive	Ginger (plus zinc)
	Moderate	Acupuncture, magnesium, osteopathic manipulation
	Low	St. John's wort, cinnamon
Migraine prevention	Supportive	Butterbur, riboflavin, magnesium
	Moderate	CoQ10
Nausea	Supportive	Ginger (pregnancy), hypnotherapy, acupuncture
Neck pain	Supportive	Acupuncture, massage
	Moderate	Chiropractic manipulation, Alexander technique
Oral/dental health	Moderate	Probiotics
Pain (chronic)	Supportive	Mind-body, meditation, yoga, biofeedback, acupuncture
	Moderate	Hypnotherapy, electromagnetic therapy
	Low	Reiki, reflexology, Feldenkrais, low-level light therapy, homeopathy, aromatherapy
Parkinson's disease	Supportive	Music therapy
	Moderate	Massage
	Low	CoQ10, ashwagandha
Pediatrics	Moderate	Hypnotherapy, massage
	Low	Osteopathic manipulation
Post-traumatic stress disorder	Supportive	Guided imagery
	Moderate	Yoga, hypnotherapy
Psychiatric disorders	Supportive	Music therapy
	Low	Meditation
Sexual function	Moderate	Ginseng

Condition or Focus	Evidence*	Methods or supplements
Sleep disorders (not insomnia)	Supportive	Music therapy, melatonin (jet lag)
	Moderate	Meditation
	Low	St. John's wort, essential oils
Smoking cessation	Supportive	Mind-body, yoga, meditation
	Moderate	Guided imagery, massage
	Low	Acupuncture, biofeedback, hypnotherapy
Stress	Supportive	Acupuncture, tai chi, qi gong, meditation, yoga, massage, guided imagery, hypno- therapy
	Low	Reiki, reflexology, Feldenkrais
Stroke recovery	Supportive	Biofeedback, guided imagery, mind-body
	Moderate	Traditional Chinese medicine, acupuncture, music therapy
Substance abuse	Supportive	Mind-body
	Moderate	Meditation, guided imagery
	Low	Acupuncture
Temporomandibular joint (TMJ) **symptoms**	Supportive	Biofeedback, mind-body
	Moderate	Hypnotherapy
Tinnitus	Supportive	Mind-body
	Low	Biofeedback, ginkgo
Vertigo	Moderate	Homeopathy, ginkgo
Weight management	Moderate	Guided imagery, hypnotherapy, yoga, mind-body, mindfulness
	Low	Meditation

*Supportive evidence includes strong evidence of effectiveness or mostly supportive evidence. Moderate evidence includes good evidence but also may include a significant number of stud- ies that are weak, ambiguous, or weak in evidence. Low evidence includes mostly weak, equiv- ocal, or negative studies that have not demonstrated effectiveness.

Glossary

Acute

Sudden or rapid, as in acute muscle cramps that can occur with vigorous exercise.

Adaptogen

General term for a therapy or substance that fortifies the body's ability to cope with physical or mental stress; may also boost overall energy levels or heighten the sense of well-being.

Allopath/allopathic

A term coined by the father of homeopathy, Samuel Hahnemann, to refer to practices or methods to treat disease that counterbalance or produce effects opposite to the disease, as with using antibiotics to combat an infection. A contrasting viewpoint from homeopathy, used today to refer to conventional or mainstream medicine or its practitioners, or by osteopaths in referring to M.D.s.

Antioxidant

A molecule or substance that quenches or neutralizes reactive forms of oxygen and other molecules known as **free radicals**, which are formed as cells transfer electron particles among sugars, amino acids, and other molecules. Antioxidants may sometimes switch their mode of action and instead become pro-oxidants that cause the formation of free radicals. Antioxidant balance plays an important yet elusive role in states of disease and health.

Alternative medicine

Medical beliefs or practices that were not classically taught, accepted, or practiced at mainstream medical institutions that may include unproven approaches to health. When used, alternative approaches may be used in place of conventional care. Because of increasing acceptance and widespread use of many practices formerly considered "alternative" that do not exclude mainstream care and that are now part of contemporary care, this term is losing favor.

Bioavailability

With respect to dietary supplements, the proportion or amount of an ingested product that is absorbed by the body and available for the body to use or store.

Bioenergetics

Healing approaches that seek to enhance, restore, or rebalance the body's inner energy; sometimes called energy therapies.

Biofield

A force or combination of forces—such as electromagnetic fields associated with living things—that may be modified as part of a healing therapy or that may be affected at a distance or by certain actions; Reiki and healing touch are examples of biofield therapies.

Cardioprotection

Therapies, actions, or activities that protect heart cells, tissues, or function from injury due to any number of causes.

Cardiovascular disease

A wide-ranging group of diseases and disorders pertaining to the heart and/or the blood vessels of the heart, the blood vessels supplying the brain (cerebrovascular), the arms or legs (peripheral vascular disease), and/or diseases or conditions of clotting within veins that may travel to distant sites—as in deep venous thrombosis (in the legs) or pulmonary embolism (clots that travel to the lungs from another site, for example, the pelvis or legs); sometimes abbreviated CVD.

Chronic

Persisting over time, as in a chronic condition that lasts for a few months or years. Chronic symptoms may reach a plateau, without significant change or improvement. Chronic pain is defined as pain lasting longer than 12 weeks.

Complementary medicine

Therapies, beliefs, or practices that fall outside of classically mainstream medical beliefs or practices but are generally used alongside conventional care; may be abbreviated together with alternative medicine as CAM.

Controlled trial or study

A study of a treatment or intervention that divides the subjects into treatment and nontreatment groups to study the possible effects of an intervention. The value and evidence grading of a controlled trial depends in part on the size of the population under study (bigger is usually better), whether or not the investigators and the subjects knew which group was receiving the therapy and how that "double-blinding" was done, and whether or not the subjects in the different groups were selected or assigned at random (randomized controlled trial).

Dietary supplement

In the U.S., a product containing a single dietary ingredient or combination of dietary ingredients taken in the diet and meant to supplement or add nutritional value to the diet. Dietary supplement ingredients include vitamins, minerals, herbs or other botanicals, amino acids, enzymes, and—rarely—hormones (DHEA). Dietary supplements are regulated more like foods than drugs and are not tested by the Food and Drug Administration for efficacy or safety before being sold.

Essential nutrients

Nutrients that cannot be made within the body and that must be supplied by the diet; omega-3 fatty acids are examples of essential fatty acids.

Evidence-based approach

A nonintuitive decision-making policy or practice that attempts to harmonize the best scientific practices from literature with the skills and knowledge of the practitioner, combined with the beliefs and preferences of the patient, to develop a care plan. Scientific literature may be graded for the strength of the evidence it presents depending on the study group size, statistics, study design, interpretation, and other factors.

Free radicals

Unstable and therefore highly reactive elements and compounds that seek stability by combining with another element such as oxygen. Free radicals are formed by normal cellular processes as well as by malignant cells, or they may form as a result of exposure to certain toxic substances such as air pollution and environmental contaminants, the ultraviolet rays of sunlight, chemotherapy, smoking, intense exercise, and other factors. Free radicals have the potential for damage and healing as part of the body's internal defense system, making balance essential. Free radicals are deactivated by antioxidants.

GI

Gastrointestinal, usually referring to the stomach and intestines, although the entire GI tract begins at the mouth and ends at the anus.

Herb-drug interaction

Any one or combination of many potential effects that result from combining herbal remedies alone or with prescription or over-the-counter drugs. These reactions can include toxicity, lower or higher levels of the herb/supplement or drug, specific organ damage, interference with the effectiveness of any of the agents taken (for example, the interference of St. John's wort with the effectiveness of birth control pills may lead to unwanted pregnancy), reactions, or other effects.

Holistic (or wholistic)

Involving the whole person beyond merely his or her physical self, including emotional, mental, spiritual, social, familial, occupational, environmental, or other aspects of being.

Integrative medicine

A comprehensive approach to health and healing that brings together conventional, complementary, and nonconventional practices in an evidence-informed, collaborative way that may include or accommodate many different types of disciplines and beliefs for the benefit of the patient.

Mainstream medicine

Medical practices or beliefs typically associated with conventional Western medical care as taught at most American medical schools and as commonly practiced by such graduates; also called conventional, allopathic, Western, or technology-based medicine.

Mind-body practices

Methods and practices that use the power of the mind to positively influence well-being or health; examples include meditation, guided imagery, and other relaxation therapies.

Mortality

The death rate, as in "all-cause mortality," in which the death rate from all causes combined was considered or calculated.

Musculoskeletal

The bony and soft tissues and structures that make up, surround, and support the skeleton, including bones, cartilage, joints, muscles, fascia, ligaments, and tendons.

Neuroprotection

Protection of brain or nerve cells, tissues, or function from injury due to any number of causes.

Observational trial or study

In humans, a scientific study that looks at populations or groups of people to determine whether an association exists between the treatment under study (for example, an herb, vitamin, diet, or exercise program) and the risk of a disease or condition; does not prove cause and effect.

Phytochemicals

Natural and bioactive chemicals that are present within plants or botanical products made from plants; antioxidants and polyphenols are examples of phytochemicals.

Phytonutrients

Phytochemicals that have a nutritional action or value, usually referring to actions in humans.

TCM

A common abbreviation for traditional Chinese medicine.

Topical

Applied to a surface of the body such as the skin or the inside of the mouth.

Traditional medicine

Healing practices associated with any of the ancient, traditional, or whole systems of care such as Ayurveda, traditional Chinese medicine, Navajo medicine, and other folk-, tribal- or culture-based remedies and beliefs.

Index